AN INTRODUCTION TO BEHAVIOURAL SCIENCE AND DENTISTRY

AN INTRODUCTION TO BEHAVIOURAL SCIENCE & DENTISTRY

DAVID LOCKER

TAVISTOCK/ROUTLEDGE

First published 1989
by Routledge
11 New Fetter Lane, London EC4P 4EE
29 West 35th Street, New York, NY 10001

Typeset by Pat and Anne Murphy,
Highcliffe-on-Sea, Dorset
Printed in Great Britain

British Library Cataloguing in Publication Data

Locker, David
An introduction to behavioural science and dentistry.
1. Dentistry. Applications of behavioural sciences
I. Title
617.6

ISBN 0-415-01826-9

Contents

For
R.N.H., D.C.K. and J.F.

Introduction

Twenty years ago, it was uncommon for dental students to be given lectures on topics drawn from the behavioural sciences. Then the undergraduate curriculum was certainly less crowded and arguably less sophisticated in its approach to patient care. Since then, it has been realized that interpersonal skills are as essential to dental practice as the clincial and technical skills that are the main focus of dental education. At the very least, the dental practitioner needs to know something about the sociology and psychology of pain and the behavioural responses of patients to dental treatment. The behavioural sciences courses that are now becoming a component of undergraduate education aim to provide the student with a basic understanding of these issues and their implications for the effective practice of dentistry.

This book takes a somewhat broader view and discusses a wider range of issues relevant to the provision of dental health care. A number of contemporary trends, already beginning to have some impact on the form and content of dental practice, means that these issues are as relevant to dentistry as they are to medicine. These trends include changes in the pattern of dental and oral disease; changes in dental practice organization and methods of paying the dentist; more knowledgeable consumers of health services who demand high quality personal and technical care; threats to professional autonomy and monopoly by para-professional occupations, governments, and third party payers; an increasing emphasis on the disabling and handicapping effects of oral disease and the emergence of psychosocial therapies for patients with chronic facial pain disorders. These trends, and their effects, demand a broad understanding of the origins and distribution of oral disease and the social context within which dentistry is practised.

The book has been based on a series of lectures given to second- and third-year students in the undergraduate dental programme at the University of Toronto by staff in the Department of Community Dentistry. Although predominantly sociological in approach, it draws on sociology, psychology, epidemiology, and clinical dentistry as appropriate. The book is not a comprehensive review of the literature on behavioural science and dentistry. Such a review is to be found in Cohen and Bryant (1984) — see 'Further reading', p. 235. Rather, its aim is to provide a concise introduction to a wide range of topics and issues relevant to the dental practitioner and the practice of dentistry. These issues have been selected on the basis of personal interest and preference, and many topics which could, and perhaps should, have been included have not been addressed. For this reason, the book does not stand alone and should be used in conjunction with a course of lectures and classes which fill in the gaps and provide more a detailed discussion than has been feasible here. In fact, the book was written so that the relatively few hours devoted to the teaching of the behavioural sciences need not be taken up in giving students basic information, but can be used to explore in more depth than would otherwise be possible the issues raised and their implications for the practice of dentistry.

The book consists of three sections. Chapters 1 to 6 are concerned with the relationship between social and psychological factors and oral disease. They examine both the role of such factors in the onset of disease and the social and psychological consequences of such disorders. Chapters 8 to 12 cover the sociology and psychology of dental practice and focus predominantly on the patient–practitioner relationship. Traditional psychological topics such as pain and anxiety are included since these are seen as features of the patient–practitioner relationship and not characteristics of individuals. Chapter 7, which examines illness behaviour and the seeking of dental health care, links these two major areas of inquiry. Finally, Chapters 13 to 15 raise some of the social and political issues surrounding the health care professions and the provision of health services.

Although the book is about dentistry, extensive use has been made of research and literature on sociology and medical care. There are two reasons for this. First, some important issues have been inadequately investigated in dentistry. The study of the dentist–patient relationship, for example, is nowhere near as advanced as the study of the doctor–patient relationship. Second, the distinction between dentistry and medicine is somewhat artificial and each has much to learn from the other. For students who wish to undertake further reading, a short list of recommended texts has been included at the end of the book. Some of these are books on psychology written specifically for dental students, while others are more comprehensive texts that provide more extensive discussions of key issues. Behavioural science texts written for medical students and a book meant to be used in undergraduate sociology courses are also listed. Together they provide access to an expanding field in research and health care practice.

1

Changing patterns of disease

The patterns of death and disease affecting human populations do not remain static but change in line with social and economic development. This chapter examines changes in general and dental health, and attempts to identify the social, economic, and environmental factors responsible for the improvements in health observed over the last 150 years. This is a timely exercise, given the rapid and dramatic changes taking place in the oral health of modern populations.

A useful point of departure is the concept of the health field (Lalonde 1974). This states that any health problem can be explained in terms of human biology, the environment, lifestyle, and health care organization. These factors interact in complex ways to determine the level of health of a population. There is currently a debate over the relative significance of each in explaining historical changes in health. This is particularly the case with respect to the role of the formal health care system. Some have argued that the development of the health care professions, the growth of hospitals, and the expansion of medical knowledge which began in the middle of the nineteenth century had a major impact on health, while others argue that improvements in health can be traced to changes in society itself.

Human society and patterns of disease

Documenting historical changes in the patterns of death and disease in human populations can be a hazardous enterprise and, for want of hard evidence, must often be based on speculation.

However, it is generally agreed that human societies have passed through three major epochs, each characterized by a particular form of society and specific patterns of death and disease (McKeown 1979). Each of these types of society persist in parts of the world today.

In the *pre-agricultural epoch* human society took the form of small nomadic groups of hunter-gatherers. The necessity of following game and foraging for food meant that there was little in the way of permanent settlement. Archeological evidence suggests that life expectancy was short and mortality rates high. Because population densities were too low to support infectious disease most deaths would have been the product of violence, environmental hazards and malnutrition.

After 10,000 BC *agricultural societies* developed. These were characterized by permanent settlement, more stable food supplies based on farming, and an increase in population densities. In these societies infectious diseases were the major causes of death. A relatively poor diet and poor sanitation led to a high degree of exposure and susceptibility to diseases such as tuberculosis, cholera, dysentery, and plague, and correspondingly high death rates. In 1348 the Black Death killed 25 per cent of the population of England.

From 1750 onwards the agricultural societies of Britain and Europe began to industrialize, a process coincident with what has been called 'the modern rise of populations' and a transformation in the nature of the diseases causing death. *Early industrial societies* were characterized not only by an increase in population, but also by the concentration of the population in towns and cities. Paradoxically, urbanization and increasing population densities were accompanied by falling mortality rates, with 60 per cent of this decline due to a reduction in deaths from infectious disease. This was not due to a spontaneous change in the virulence of infectious organisms or to the development of a natural immunity on the part of the population. Rather, it was the product of social and economic change (Fitzpatrick 1986a, Hart 1985).

By the 1930s the transformation in the causes of death was well underway. In the *modern industrial era* infectious disease is a relatively unimportant cause of death (although with the rise of AIDS it may be acquiring a new significance). Rather, chronic degenerative disorders such as heart disease, cancers, and strokes are responsible for most deaths, and non-fatal disorders such as arthritis are highly prevalent. These changes can be seen in the

Table 1.1 Standardized death rates (per million) for selected conditions: England and Wales

	1848–54	1983
Tuberculosis	2901	10
Bronchitis, pneumonia, influenza	2309	1170
Cholera	1819	>1
Prematurity, immaturity and other diseases of infancy	1221	72
Scarlet fever and diphtheria	1016	>1
Cardiovascular disease	698	3768
Cancer	307	2704

Source: Fitzpatrick 1986a

data presented in Table 1.1. Although the major cause of death in the mid-nineteenth century, tuberculosis had virtually disappeared from modern populations by 1983. The chronic diseases currently responsible for most deaths are related to aging and lifestyle and, in spite of the fact that they are more common among the poorer members of society, they are often referred to as diseases of affluence.

Improvements in health: the role of medicine

The extent of the improvement in health since the middle of the nineteenth century is evident in changes in mortality and life expectancy. In the UK mortality rates were 23 per 1000 in 1851 and 11 per 1000 in 1982. Over the same period life expectancy at birth increased from 40 to 70 years for males and from 43 to 76 years for females. Since this was coincident with the development of organized medicine and a tremendous growth in the number of hospitals and medical personnel, it is easy to conclude that the rise of health care systems was responsible for this change. However, McKeown (1979) has challenged this argument on two grounds. First, he pointed out that medicine had very few effective remedies at its disposal prior to 1930, and for most of the nineteenth century unhygienic conditions and the ignorance of asepsis meant that patients entering hospital were as likely to die of hospital-acquired infections as they were of the disease that led to their admission. Second, by careful historical analysis, McKeown showed that the decline in mortality from infectious diseases began, and was almost complete, prior to the development of knowledge of the microbiological origins of these diseases or the development of effective remedies or preventive procedures. The evidence used to support this claim in the case of tuberculosis is presented in Figure 1.1. This graph shows that the decline in mortality was underway prior to the discovery of the tubercle bacillus and well before the discovery of chemotherapy or the widespread use of BCG vaccination. Most of the other major infectious diseases, such as scarlet fever, pneumonia, bronchitis, and whooping cough, show the same pattern. The only exception to this is smallpox, which declined following the discovery of vaccination against the disease.

Figure 1.1 Pulmonary tuberculosis: annual death rates for England and Wales

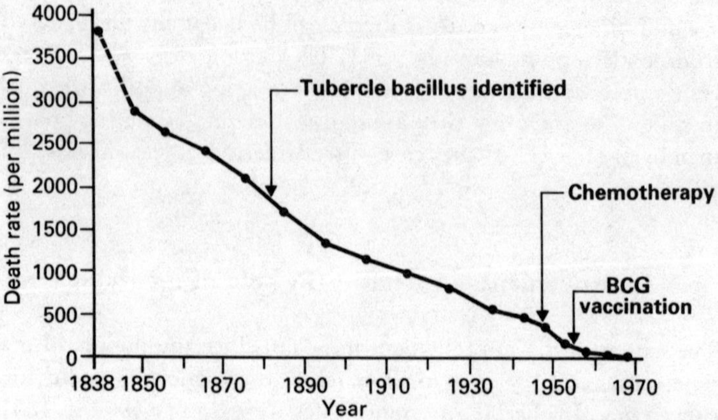

Source: McKeown 1979

McKeown's original analysis was based on data for England and Wales. He also examined data from other European countries and again concluded that factors other than medical intervention were responsible for the decline in mortality during the eighteenth and nineteenth centuries. McKinlay and McKinlay (1977) have undertaken a similar analysis using US data for the period 1900 to 1973 and shown that a substantial decline in mortality rates had occurred prior to any significant spending on health care (see Figure 1.2). The explanation favoured by these investigators is that improvements in health were the product of rising standards

Figure 1.2 Age- and sex-adjusted mortality rates for the United States (1900 – 73) (including and excluding eleven major infectious diseases) contrasted with the proportion of Gross National Product expended on medical care

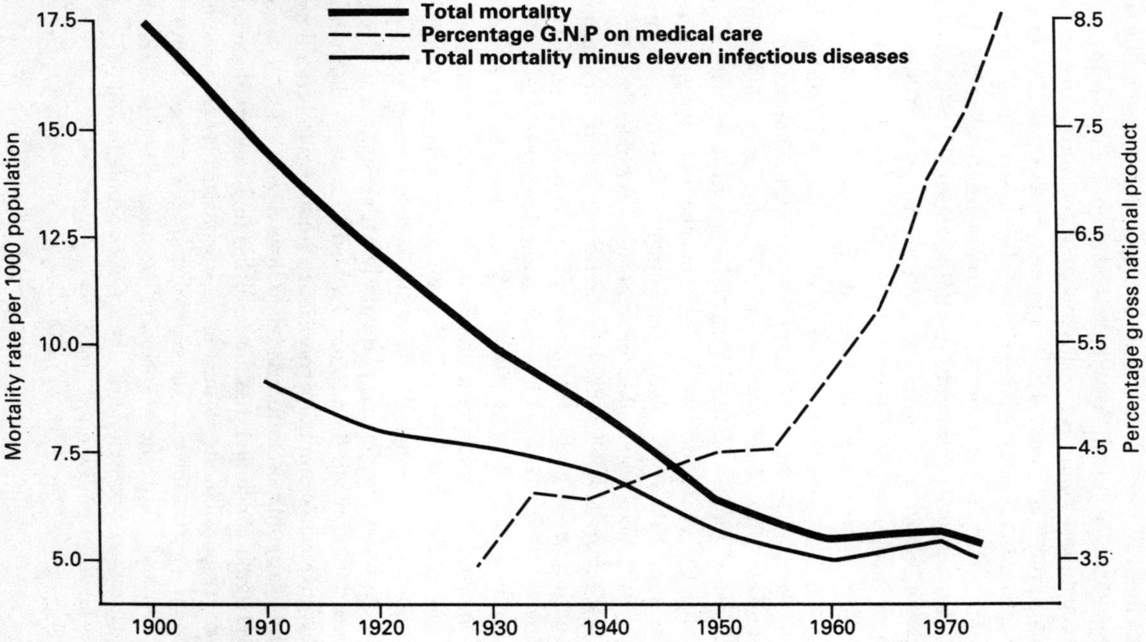

Source: McKinlay and McKinlay 1977

of living brought about by social and economic development. McKeown considered three factors to have had the greatest impact on improvements in health: diet, standards of sanitation and hygiene, and a reduction in birth rates and family size following the widespread adoption of contraception.

The nutritional status of the population of Britain improved considerably as a result of the agricultural revolution of the eighteenth century. This increased domestic productivity enormously and, combined with a more efficient means of distribution, gave the population more and better food to eat. Improved nutrition reduced deaths from starvation but, more importantly, improved host resistance to infectious disease. During the nineteenth century environmental improvements brought about by the public health movement improved the disposal of human waste and ensured a pure water supply. Along with improvements in food hygiene, this reduced the risk of exposure to water- and food-borne infectious disease. A deliberate reduction in family size by the use of contraception meant that the population did not outstrip the food supply (which was already growing due to declining death rates), eliminated infanticide, and reduced maternal and infant mortality rates (since parity — the number of births per woman — is strongly related to both). Accordingly, McKeown contends that the influences responsible for improvements in health, in order of their historical appearance and their overall effect, were economic, environmental and behavioural. Efficacious therapies beyond the few available to the Victorian medical practitioner proliferated during the 1930s and 1940s and only then began to make an important contribution to the control of bacterial infections.

McKeown has extended this historical analysis to the health problems of the present day, and here his conclusions become somewhat controversial, particularly with respect to the legitimate role of technological medicine. Nevertheless, it is still the case that the major killers in modern societies are rooted in prevailing social and economic conditions (see Chapter 15). The relationship between health and standards of living is apparent in contemporary populations in the close association between income and health (see Chapter 3), the relationship between health and unemployment, and the association between lifestyle and chronic disease. As a consequence, these health problems will not be solved by medical intervention alone.

Changing patterns of oral disease

Historical changes in dental health are more difficult to document than changes in general health. Since the mid-nineteenth century reasonably reliable statistics on death and the cause of death have been compiled and are readily available. Although some fairly crude data on dental health date back to the 1850s, systematic data were not collected until the 1920s, and regular population-based surveys did not begin to appear until the 1950s and 1960s. Even recent changes in the prevalence and distribution of dental caries are difficult to describe accurately, due to limitations in available survey data. Consequently, there remains some doubt about the extent and timing of those changes.

Archeological evidence confirms that both dental caries and periodontal disease have been present throughout the course of human history. Skulls from as long ago as the neolithic period have been found to contain teeth showing evidence of decay. However, for much of human history, the prevalence of caries has remained relatively low. During the pre-agricultural period diets were largely non-cariogenic and caries relatively minimal. Changes in diet associated with the development of agricultural societies did not result in a marked increase in caries incidence. Up to 1500 AD diets were coarse and abrasive, and produced marked attrition of the occlusal surfaces of the teeth. Consequently, coronal caries was uncommon, with the few lesions that occurred affecting the neck or root of the tooth. After 1500, however, the diets became increasingly refined, pit and fissure caries and decay of the interproximal surfaces appeared, and the prevalence of caries began to increase rapidly. However, the most dramatic increase occurred around 1850, at a time of rapid industrialization. This coincided with a significant rise in the per capita consumption of sugar and the greater processing of foods, which also increased the cariogenicity of the diet (Hardwick 1960). A similar process can be observed in many developing countries, where urbanization and a shift to a western, highly refined diet have resulted in an increase in caries rates among the more affluent members of the community. By the latter half of the century, dental caries had become established as a disease of endemic proportions and rates of tooth loss were high. These high levels of decay and tooth loss continued for the first half of the twentieth century, although tooth loss has declined since the Second World War and rates of dental caries in children have declined significantly over the last ten to twenty years. These contemporary changes have coincided with changes in dental practice, with the main orientation moving from extraction to restoration and, subsequently, to the prevention of dental disease.

Contemporary changes in oral health

Tooth loss

When describing trends in the oral health status of a population it is necessary to distinguish between changes in the prevalence of disease and changes in modes of treating disease. This distinction is most important when considering rates of tooth loss, for the interaction of these two factors is responsible for the high rates of edentulism observed in elderly people, many of whom will have lost many if not most of their teeth during the years prior to the 1940s, when extraction was the treatment of choice (Murray 1983). This means that a reduction in tooth loss over time is not necessarily indicative of a decline in the prevalence of dental disease since a change in the pattern of treatment would have the same effect. International comparisons have revealed discrepancies between the prevalence of edentulism and dental caries experience. Cohen (1978) found that the prevalence of edentulism among 35-to 44-year-olds was 6 per cent in Norway and 36 per cent in New Zealand, even though these countries had similar adult DMFT levels. This difference in rates is the product of culture and differences in attitudes towards dental treatment (Davis 1981).

A comparison of data from studies undertaken in the 1920s with data taken from studies of the 1960s and 1970s suggests that the prevalence of dental caries did not change substantially in either children or adults over this period. Table 1.2 compares the condition of specific teeth in British schoolchildren in 1925 and 1973. In 1925 62 per cent of lower first molars in 13-year-olds were decayed or missing due to caries. In 1973 80 per cent of these teeth in this age group were decayed, missing or filled. Although these statistics are not exactly comparable, they provide no evidence of a decline in caries rates over the period involved. Burt (1978) reviewed a number of studies of young adults in the US and found little variation in caries rates over a 40-year period. In a study of 12,000 employees of the Metropolitan Life Insurance Company undertaken in the 1930s, those aged 20 to 24 years had a DMFT of

Table 1.2 Comparison of the condition of specific teeth in British school children, 1925 and 1973

		Medical Research Council Survey 1925	National Survey 1973
Tooth type	Age	% Decayed[1]	% DMF[2]
Upper first molars	9	33	50
Upper first molars	13	52	78
Lower first molars	9	45	50
Lower first molars	13	62	80

1 Includes missing due to decay but not filled
2 Includes decayed, missing and filled teeth

Source: Burt 1978. Adapted

14.0 (Hollander and Dunning 1939). The National Health Examination Survey of 1960–2 found that DMFT scores for this age group were still 14.0 (Graves and Stamm 1985).

A major change in oral health status which was taking place during this period of stable caries prevalence rates was a reduction in the number of teeth lost as a result of dental disease. This is reflected in data on changes in rates of edentulism since the 1950s (see Table 1.3) and the decline in the M or missing component of DMFT scores since the 1960s (Graves and Stamm 1985). In 1960–2, 36 per cent of DMFT scores in 18- to 24-year-olds were missing teeth compared with 17 per cent in 1971–4. The most important factors responsible were changes in dental practice and the emergence of more positive attitudes towards the retention of natural teeth. These changes involved a shift in emphasis from the extraction of decayed teeth to their restoration.

Burt (1978) considers that the demise of the theory of focal infection had an important influence on approaches to dental practice. This theory, which was at its height between 1918 and the late 1940s, suggested that even mildly decayed teeth could be repositories of infection and the cause of more widespread systemic disorders. The theory was eventually discarded following the work of Easlick in 1951, but only after it had provided the rationale for the wholesale extraction of teeth. Many older people will have lost teeth not because they could not be restored, but because of a misguided effort to alleviate or avoid more general physical complaints.

Table 1.3 Percent edentulous by year and age: US adult population

Year	Age	% Edentulous	Age 65–74 % Edentulous
1957–58	All ages	13.0	55.4
1960–62	18–74	17.0	49.4
1971	All ages	11.2	45.2
1971–74	18–74	14.7	
	6–74	10.7	45.5
1976	5–70	13.0	39.7
1977	All ages	7.5	36.6
1980	All ages	8.3	33.8

Source: Weintraub and Burt 1985. Compiled from various local and national surveys

Murray (1983) has identified a number of other factors which facilitated this shift from extraction to restoration. One was the development of high speed rotary cutting instruments which revolutionized restorative treatment, enabling complex procedures, including crowns and bridgework, to be undertaken quickly and with relatively little discomfort to patients. Developments in materials and techniques also allowed teeth largely destroyed by decay to be retained instead of being removed.

Another factor which transformed dental practice was the growth in dental manpower and a reduction in dentist–population ratios. The number of dental practitioners in England and Wales grew from 9,359 in 1955 to 13,039 in 1980. A more rapid increase took place in Canada, which now has almost as many dentists serving a population of approximately half the size. In the US, however, dentist–population ratios were very favourable in 1930 and have remained more or less stable over time. Murray (1983) suggests that a low dentist–population ratio enables more time to be spent on the restoration of teeth and leads to a decline in the rate of extractions. Support for this argument is to be found in the close association between edentulism rates and dentist–population ratios. Edentulism rates are high in the UK but low in the US where utilization rates are the same but where there are almost twice as many dentists per unit population. Similarly, the regional maldistribution of dentists in the UK matches quite closely the regional differences in edentulousness.

Economic and social factors have also played an important role in the greater propensity of dentists to restore teeth. Rising levels of affluence in the US following the Second World War enabled many more people to opt for restoration rather than extraction, and the inclusion of dentistry in the National Health Service meant that the economic barriers to restorative care were removed for the British population. More recent evidence has confirmed that the cost of dental care influences the volume and complexity of care provided to the patient (see Chapter 14). Along with rising affluence, attitudes towards dental care and the natural dentition have changed, with fewer people likely to regard the loss of teeth as a natural and inevitable state of affairs. In 1968 only 27 per cent of dentate adults in Britain found the idea of having to wear full dentures upsetting; by 1978 this had risen to 48 per cent (Todd and Walker 1980).

The fairly dramatic changes in dental practice brought about by these factors is evident in data released by the Dental Estimates Board, which administers dental treatment under the National Health Service. In 1950 only 27 per cent of the fees paid by the NHS to dentists were for restoration, crowns, bridges and root canal therapy. The comparable figure for 1980 was 49 per cent. A comparison of the volume of treatments provided in 1970 and 1980 show that this trend is continuing. Over this short period of time the number of teeth extracted fell by 40 per cent, the provision of crowns increased by 380 per cent and deep scalings and periodontal surgery increased by 1600 per cent. In 1980, only 6 per cent of expenditures on the dental care of children were for the extraction of teeth.

Dental caries

The above analysis suggests that early improvements in oral health status were due to technological, economic and attitudinal factors and their impact on treatment patterns. More recently observed changes consist of a decline in the prevalence and severity of dental disease, particularly among children and young adults, and are the result of a different set of influences.

The most startling and largely unanticipated change in the oral health status of modern populations has been the substantial reduction in the decay experience of children. This has been observed in eight developed countries and, despite variation in populations and methods, the data indicate an overall reduction of between 30 and 50 per cent over the past 10 to 20 years. In the US the interpretation of epidemiological data collected during the 1970s suggests that the rate fell by 36 per cent in that decade alone (Burt 1985). A similar reduction occurred in British schoolchildren over more or less the same period (Anderson 1981, Anderson *et al.* 1981).

In most of the countries reporting a decline the following trends are apparent: 1) this relatively sharp decline has occurred in both primary and permanent dentitions; 2) the percentage of caries-free children has increased dramatically, so that about 60 per cent of decay now occurs in about 20 per cent of children; 3) the decline has occurred in non-fluoridated as well as fluoridated communities; 4) the most noticeable reduction has been on smooth and interproximal surfaces, but substantial declines have been reported for pit and fissure surfaces; 5) significant reductions have been observed over periods of time as short as 3 to 5 years (Graves *et al.* 1986). For example, studies of five-year-old children in both fluoridated and non-fluoridated communities in the north of England show that the percentage of children who were caries-free increased from 34 to 55 per cent and from 12 to 31 per cent respectively between 1976 and 1981 (Carmichael *et al.* 1980).

The implications of this decline in childhood caries for the practice of dentistry are as yet unclear. How the trend will develop is not known with any certainty, nor is it known whether the relative absence of dental caries among contemporary child populations will continue into adulthood and old age. It has been suggested that current trends may represent a delay in onset and not a lifetime of freedom from the disease. An explanation of the decline in caries and identification of the social, environmental, or other factors responsible would make it possible to project caries experience in the future. This is not an easy task, given the number of factors which could be involved. Moreover, the relative contribution of these factors is difficult to assess unless the date of onset of the decline is known.

Although reductions in caries prevalence were first documented in the late 1970s, it is clear that the decline began much earlier. Burt (1985) has re-evaluated data from studies dating back to the late 1940s and finds that caries was actively declining during the 1960s but could possibly have begun to do so soon after the Second World War. This suggestion is based on data collected as part of the first fluoridation project in Grand Rapids, Michigan. This showed that mean deft and DMFT scores for the control (non-fluoridated) community of Muskegon fell by 1.5 to 4.5 per cent between the baseline examinations in 1944–5 and the follow-up examinations in 1949–50. Reductions as high as 22 per cent were observed in some age groups over this five-year period. However, as Burt notes, these differences could be methodological in origin and may not be documenting a real decline. Given that control groups used in other fluoridation projects showed no such reduction over the same time period the Muskegon data must be viewed with some caution.

Data from Ontario, Canada, give a clearer indication that the reduction in caries experience did not start until the beginning of the 1960s (see Figure 1.3). The Ontario data suggest that dental caries increased in prevalence during the 1950s, a trend also observed in some European countries following the end of war-time food rationing and the greater availability of sugar. The mean deft/DMFT scores and the percentage of children with some experience of decay peak around 1960 for all age groups, following which they show a systematic and continuous decline (Johnston *et al.* 1986). As in the US, there remain regional differences throughout Ontario and it seems reasonable to suggest that the trend was not necessarily uniform across communities but may well have occurred first in those with the most favourable caries experience. It is certainly the case that the rate of decline is two to three times more rapid in those areas where the rates of decay were already low.

Clearly, it is difficult, if not impossible, to be precise about the beginning of the decline in caries rates. Consequently, it is even more difficult to assess the relative contribution of the factors that are used to explain this decline. Many such factors may have played an important role. Whether one factor was largely responsible, whether it was a combination of factors, or whether the decline is due to factors not yet identified is unknown (Johnston *et al.* 1986). The main contenders are water fluoridation, fluoridated toothpastes, changes in levels of sugar consumption, vitamin enrichment of foods, improved oral hygiene, the widespread use of antibiotics, and the reduction in unfilled cavities. Some of these constitute intrinsic factors, reducing the susceptibility of teeth to attack by cariogenic micro-organisms and others are extrinsic, modifying the oral environment.

Fluoridation of water supplies has been the main and most successful strategy in the prevention of dental decay. Water fluoridation began in 1945, and by 1980 approximately half of the population of the US were receiving fluoridated water. In Canada

Figure 1.3 *Mean decayed, filled and missing teeth per child by age and survey year: Ontario, Canada*

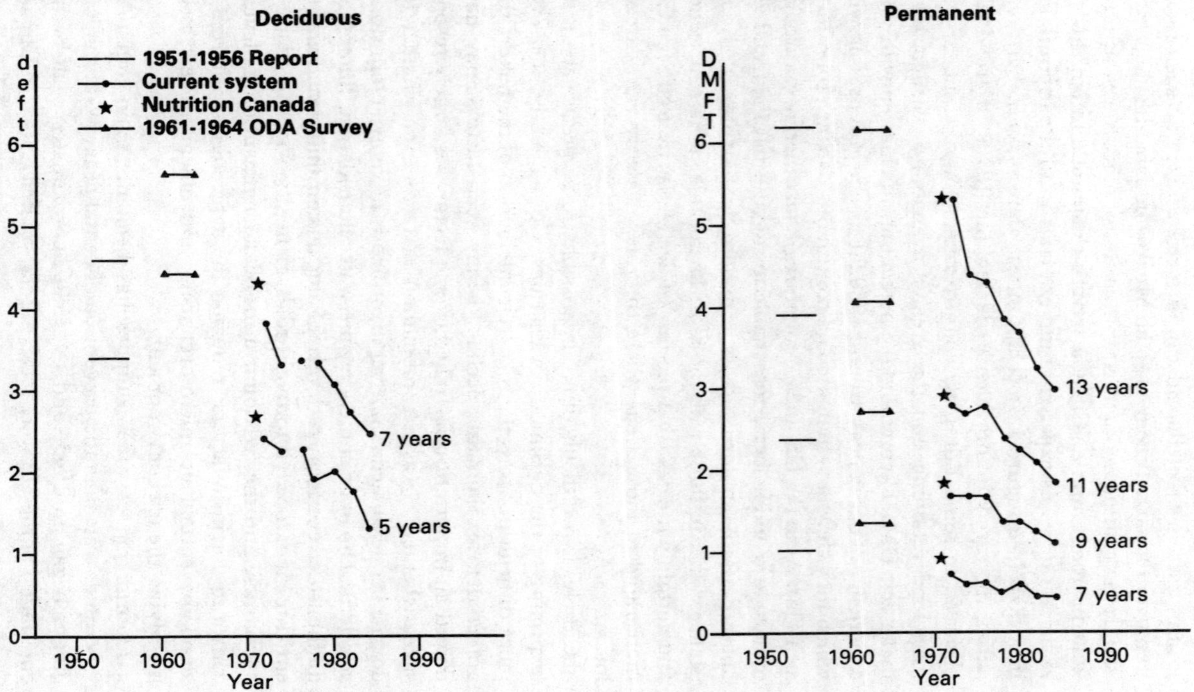

Source: Johnston *et al.* 1986. Compiled from various surveys

the percentage varies by province, from a high of 65 in Manitoba to a low of 9 in Newfoundland. In the UK, the proportion of the population drinking fluoridated water is low — less than 10 per cent receive fluoride in this way. While fluoridated water has been responsible for a decline of 50 per cent in dental caries rates in the communities covered, it cannot explain the contemporary reduction in dental decay in all children. The reason for this is that the decline has been observed in non-fluoridated as well as fluoridated communities and is of a similar magnitude in both. Moreover, in many fluoridated communities decay rates were falling before the adoption of a water fluoridation programme (Diesendorf 1986).

Jackson (1987) has examined the claim that fluoridated toothpastes have played a major role in reducing dental caries, particularly in populations without the benefit of fluoridated water. Clinical trials of fluoridated toothpastes have produced reductions in caries increments of 0 to 50 per cent, with an average of 24 per cent. Five comparable trials carried out in the UK produced a reduction of only 8 per cent in children aged 11 to 14 years. Given that these results were obtained under the cushioned circumstances of clinical trials, it is unlikely that an effect of this magnitude would have been produced under real life circumstances. Investigators in the US and Europe have found reductions in dental decay far beyond those which could be expected even if the effect of fluoride toothpastes was equivalent to that seen under experimental conditions. Jackson also presents data to show that sales of fluoride toothpastes only began in quantity in the 1970s, some ten years after the decline in caries seems to have begun (see Figure 1.4). Accordingly they could have had no influence on the initiation of this decline. Subsequently, he examined the hypothesis that the preventive effect of these toothpastes accelerated the fall in the prevalence of decay. Again, the magnitude of the change in prevalence rates during this period was too great to be attributed to toothpastes.

Since sugar consumption is a major determinant of the level of caries in a community, a reduction in sugar consumption might explain the decline in dental decay. Although changes in the consumption of sugars and processed foods have been associated with rises and falls in caries rates in the past, there is no convincing evidence that contemporary declines are the product of less sugar in the diet. Data from the US indicate that the average per capita consumption of sugar increased between 1962 and 1971 and has

Figure 1.4 *Mean DMF values of five-year-old English schoolchildren from non-fluoridated communities, 1947–80, together with UK sales of fluoridated toothpastes*

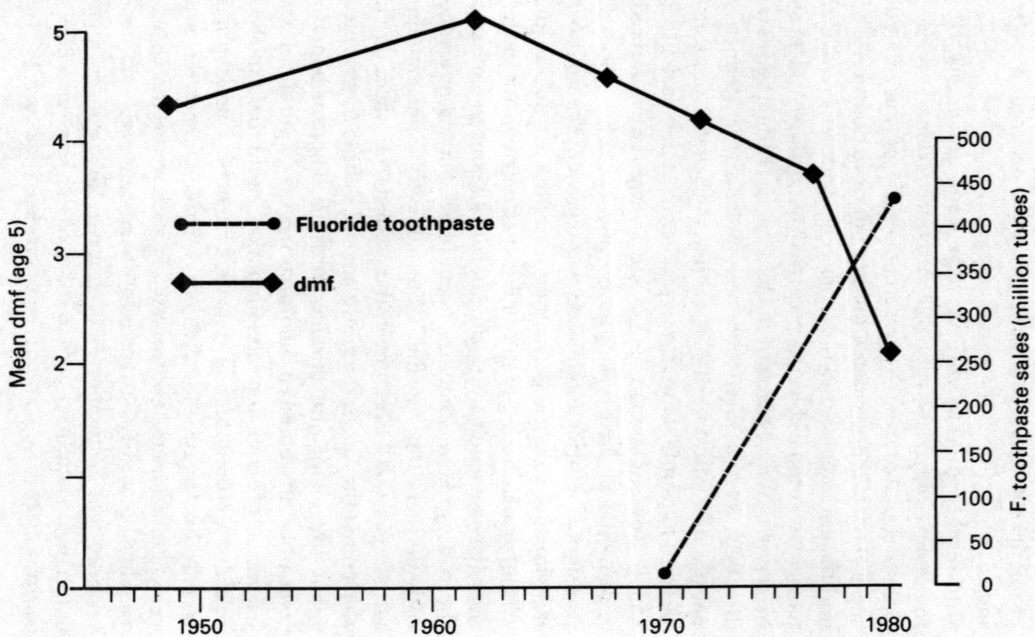

Source: Jackson 1987

remained stable since then. Data from Finland show the same kind of trend (Tala and Ainamo 1982); in Finland candy consumption increased five-fold between 1920 and 1978. There have, however, been changes in the type of sugar eaten and in its pattern of consumption. Since the 1960s the consumption of sucrose has fallen and that of fructose increased, largely because of the greater use of the latter in food manufacturing. However, since recent evidence suggests that both are metabolized by acid-producing bacteria, the implications of this change are unclear. A second trend which may be of relevance is the increasing consumption of sugars in the form of soft drinks rather than confectionery. This probably indicates an increased frequency of sugar consumption — the critical factor with respect to decay — and, if accurate, should increase rather than decrease caries prevalence rates.

Trends in gingivitis and studies of oral hygiene both lend support to the idea that oral health care behaviours have improved and the amounts of debris and plaque in mouths reduced. This is particularly marked among children and young adults, but has been noted in longitudinal studies of older populations (Douglass *et al.* 1983). Even though formal health education programmes have not proved to be effective other than in the short term, there does seem to be a greater awareness of the need for and value of oral health care among all sections of the population. However, oral hygiene plays a far less significant role in caries than it does in periodontal disease and it is unlikely that it has contributed much to declining caries rates in young children.

The remaining explanatory factors suggest a change in the frequency of infection with those oral micro-organisms implicated in the caries process. One such factor is the increase in the utilization of dentists and a reduction in the number of cavities which provide locations for colonization by cariogenic bacteria. It has been suggested that increases in the use of antibiotics may have suppressed levels of oral micro-organisms. There is some evidence indicating that children who take frequent courses of antibiotics experience less caries, although this could be explained by a number of confounding factors. However, despite a marked increase in the use of antibiotics in the US, the mean number of prescriptions issued per person per year is less than one. This is probably too low to have any long-term effect on oral micro-organisms. Nor is there any evidence to suggest that levels of infection with *Streptococcus mutans*, the most likely bacterial cause of caries, are falling. On the contrary, the organism appears to be endemic in young children and even when cleared from the oral cavity by anti-microbial agents, the level of reinfection is high.

The ecological theory of disease

None of the factors reviewed above offers a convincing explanation of the decline in caries among children. Claims that mass preventive measures, coupled with individual and professional preventive endeavours, have been responsible are not supported by the evidence. That such measures have had *some* influence is certain, but they do not seem to account for the *totality* of the decline observed. Even when taking all factors into account, and assuming maximum possible effects, there is an unexplained residual fall of more than 25 per cent. It is possible that it is the interaction of these factors which is responsible, each enhancing the causal role of the others. Alternatively, it may be due to none of these factors, either individually or combined, but may be the product of changes in general susceptibility to oral disease and the better adaptation of the human organism to its environment.

According to the ecological view of disease, health status is the result of the human organism's efforts to adapt to and reach a state of equilibrium with the physical and social environment. When the environment is subject to rapid change, biological and social adaptive mechanisms may fail and result in disease. Burt (1978) suggests hat the rapid environmental changes brought about by industrialization were matched by changes in diet and changes in the oral environment. An epidemic of dental caries was the outcome. From this perspective, the contemporary decline in caries among children may represent adaptation to the conditions that cause disease and the emergence of natural immunity. There are certainly other historical precedents for the decline of various diseases in populations, even in the absence of medical measures to treat them. Leprosy, for example, was a major disease in Europe during the fourteenth century but its significance diminished over time and it gradually disappeared. In modern populations certain sub-groups are more susceptible to disease than others even when exposed to the same risk factors. Diseases which initially affect the more affluent sections of the population soon become more common among the poor. In the case of dental caries, general improvements in social and economic well-being may make the individual more disease-resistant even in the face of an unfavourable diet. An explanation based on the notion of general susceptibility would also appear to be consistent with the distribution of dental caries among children; that is, a high proportion of the disease occurring in a small proportion of the population.

Clearly, there is much about the ecology of disease that is not well understood. However, if this explanation does have any merit, then children represent a new generation of individuals who are relatively immune to caries. Data on disease patterns among this and succeeding generations of children as they age will indicate whether this characterization is correct.

The future of dentistry

The lack of a precise explanation of the changes in caries prevalence among children make it difficult to predict the extent to which future generations will be affected by the disease. Burt (1985) believes that the decline in caries will continue but that caries is unlikely to disappear, at least in the near future. Johnston *et al.* (1986) used statistical techniques to fit curves to the Ontario data and to project caries prevalence to the end of the century. Their analysis indicates that the percentage of the population with caries in areas where levels are already low may be close to zero by the year 2000 and under 10 per cent throughout the remainder of the province. Such levels of disease will result in a major change in the pattern of dental practice and a significant reallocation of treatment resources. Certainly, treatment and preventive programmes will need to be directed at the minority of children who remain susceptible to high levels of caries but currently receive low levels of care (Graves *et al.* 1986).

The impact of falling caries rates among children on the future need and demand for dental services will force changes on the dental profession. One solution to the problem of reduced demand is the marketing of dental services in order to reach those with low levels of utilization. Schoen (1985) believes that this will prove to be only a temporary solution and calls for radical changes in the structure of the profession. This involves the emergence of a new non-surgical dental care provider, in the form of an expanded-duty hygienist, skilled in prevention and behaviour modification, who would offer primary care. The dentist would be a secondary provider, accepting patients only on referral, and responsible for the type of care currently offered by specialists. Drastic cuts would need to be made in the numbers trained in order to match levels of demand for these surgical services. Data on dental disease among both children and adults need to be collected in order to determine whether such radical approaches are necessary. It may be that oral disease among the increasing number of dentate elderly will mitigate the effects of improved oral health in children and ensure that the volume of treatment required in the population overall declines only marginally.

2
Psychosocial factors and dental disease

This chapter examines the role played by social and psychological factors in the onset of disease. This area of enquiry is generally referred to as *social epidemiology* or *psychosocial epidemiology*. In combination with the relatively new discipline of psychophysiology, it explores the links between the social environment, emotional states, physiological changes, and disease. Research exploring these links with respect to oral disorders has a long history. A review of the literature on stress and periodontal disease was published as early as 1947 (Miller and Firestone 1947). In that review the somewhat awkward term 'psychosomatic dentistry' was used to refer to 'the relationship between mental well-being and the integrity of the oral tissues'. Since then research has proliferated, so that a detailed review of the field published in 1984 contained references to over 400 papers (Rugh *et al.* 1984) concerned with the relationship between psychological processes and hard and soft tissue diseases. Contemporary interest, however, centres around the association between psychological stress and chronic oro-facial pain conditions.

In spite of the number of papers referenced by Rugh *et al.* (1984) in their recent review, it is clear that the research effort devoted to the psychosocial origins of oral disease is minute when compared to that invested in the investigation of physical and biological causes. There is every indication that this is beginning to change, partly in response to the current emphasis on prevention and health promotion, and partly in response to the recognition that physical and biological factors always work in combination with a variety of other causes, including social and psychological factors, to produce disease. The value of this broader view with respect to patient care is easy to demonstrate.

First, the identification of *all* the factors involved in the onset of disease provides a more comprehensive understanding of patients and their health problems; second, it offers greater scope for prevention, and third, it suggests alternative or supplementary therapies. For example, take the following hypothetical sequence of events:

1 Low income → 2 Poor housing → 3 Stress → 4 Muscle hyperactivity
↓
5 Temporomandibular joint problems

In this example, each and all of stages 1 to 4 could be considered to be causes of temporomandibular joint problems and treatment could be directed at each stage in the causal chain. Traditional therapies for TMJ problems have often been directed at symptoms rather than causes, or have been directed at the temporomandibular joint itself. Analgesics to control pain and surgical intervention to remove the head of the condular process are treatments that have been used. Increasingly, other therapies are being offered to TMJ patients. Biofeedback therapy is being used to help the patient to detect and control hyperactivity in the masticatory muscles and counselling is being used to help the patient recognize and cope with stress. Here, we are moving backwards along the causal chain in order to offer patients less invasive therapies. Theoretically, the causes of stress — bad housing and low income — could also be the target of therapies. It is not unusual, for example, for medical practitioners to assist their patients to acquire better or more appropriate accommodation in order to relieve stress and promote health.

However, the extent to which the role of social and psychological factors are acknowledged, and psychologically-based treatments are offered, depends upon our notions about the relationship between the body and the mind, and our ideas about the causes of disease. These ideas have not been stable, but have changed considerably over the course of medical history.

The development of medical science

Prior to the seventeenth century, the development of medical science was severely limited by religious beliefs which prevented the dissection of the human body. At that time, Christian doctrine viewed the body and the soul as one and the same, and demanded that the human body remained intact after death in order that the soul might ascend to heaven. This view was successfully challenged by the philosopher René Descartes, who believed that the mind and the body were independent, with the body being a mere physical entity which was activated by mental processes. The 'Cartesian revolution' which stemmed from a general acceptance of this view freed medical science from religious constraint and heralded significant discoveries in anatomy and physiology. However, this separation of mind and body also involved constraints on the development of thought about the origins of disease. Underlying much of what constitutes medical practice is an approach that has come to be called the 'biomechanical model'. Here the body is regarded as a machine which can be corrected when things go wrong by procedures designed to restore the normal functioning of its component parts. These procedures generally involve neutralizing the specific agents or modifying the physical processes responsible for the disease. This approach, along with the doctrine of specific aetiology, has meant that for much of this century clinical practice has largely ignored, if not denied, the influence of social and psychological factors in disease.

Theories of disease

The monocausal (or germ) theory of disease

Prior to the work of Pasteur and Koch, disease was attributed to spiritual forces (a punishment by God for sinful behaviour), or mechanical forces (the result of an imbalance in 'humours' or body fluids). In England and the USA, both of which experienced cholera epidemics during the early nineteenth century, cholera was ascribed to a life of vice or a weak moral character, and other diseases were ascribed to 'miasma' or bad air arising out of dirt and decaying organic matter. Although the idea that disease was caused by a transmissible agent had been expressed since the mid-sixteenth century, it was only in the latter half of the nineteenth century that it began successfully to challenge the miasma theory of disease. It was Pasteur and Koch who showed that this agent was a living organism, invisible to the naked eye, which entered the body via food, water, air or the bites of infected animals and insects. In 1882, Koch isolated and grew the bacillus responsible for tuberculosis, and between 1897 and 1900 the organisms responsible for 22 diseases were identified. From this work emerged the doctrine of specific aetiology, the idea that each disease has a single and specific cause. This doctrine has been very influential in guiding medical research and approaches to treatment over the past century. For example, a great deal of research effort is still devoted to identifying the microbiological causes of dental caries and therapeutic agents which will kill or control them.

The epidemiological triangle

The germ theory of disease seems to suggest that the introduction of an organism into a community is sufficient in and of itself to cause disease. This is clearly not the case: we are continually exposed to a wide variety of pathogens and yet rarely succumb to disease. Consequently, an agent, whether it be a micro-organism or noxious physical substance such as asbestos, cannot be considered to be '*the* cause' of a disease. From an epidemiological point of view, such an agent is a necessary but not a sufficient cause, because suitable conditions with respect to the host and the environment must be present before the disease develops (Mausner and Kramer 1985). In this respect, all diseases, including infections, are multifactorial and have multiple causes.

The epidemiological triangle sees disease arising out of an interaction between an agent, a host and the environment. Host factors may be generic or acquired (as in the development of specific immunity following immunization) and determine susceptibility to disease, while environmental factors may be biological, social or physical, and affect exposure and susceptibility. The social environment as a cause of ill health is examined in detail later in this chapter.

One of the main contributions of the epidemiological, as opposed to the clinical, approach is that there are many opportunities for promoting the health of a population other than by attacking the specific agent involved in the agent–host–environment triangle. As the last chapter demonstrated, the modification of factors which influence susceptibility and exposure was responsible for the improvements in human health which took place over the course of the nineteenth and early twentieth centuries.

The web of causation

The epidemiological triangle provides a useful explanation of the origins of infectious diseases but is less useful in aiding our understanding of chronic, degenerative disorders such as heart disease, stroke, schizophrenia and arthritis. With diseases of this type no agent has been identified which can be ascribed a causal role or targeted for eradication. In order to explain diseases of this type, MacMahon and Pugh (1970) introduced the concept of a 'web of causation'. According to this concept, diseases such as coronary heart disease develop through complex interactions of many factors which form interlocking causal chains. These factors may be biophysical, social or psychological, and may act to promote or inhibit the development of disease. For example, some of the factors implicated in heart disease are saturated fats in the diet, smoking, physical inactivity, stress, Type A personality, obesity, blood cholesterol levels, alcohol consumption, hypertension, diabetes, and the balance between high density and low density lipoproteins in the blood. Since many of these factors are susceptible to change, prevention currently offers a better route to health than cure. It should also be noted that many of the factors associated with CHD have also been identified as risk factors for other diseases, for example, stroke and lung cancer.

The theory of general susceptibility

This theory has emerged over the last ten years or so and is not concerned with identifying single or multiple risk factors involved in the onset of specific disorders. Rather, it seeks to understand why some social groups seem to be more susceptible to disease in general. For example, Table 2.1 shows that the single, widowed and divorced have consistently higher mortality rates than the married, the differences being much larger for men than for women. Such differences were first observed in 1859, confirmed in a classic study of suicide undertaken by the French sociologist

Durkheim in 1897, and are consistent across cultures, social structures and health care systems. Only a small part of the observed associations can be attributed to the selective effects of marriage or artifacts of data collection (Morgan 1980). One explanation for these differences is that marital status has an influence on psychological states and lifestyles, which are, in turn, related to the risk of disease. Some support for this has been presented by Gove (1979) who showed that differences in mortality by marital status were largest for those conditions in which such factors are believed to play a prominent role. For example, the rates for suicide, lung cancer, cirrhosis of the liver, tuberculosis and diabetes are from one-and-a-half to nine times as high among the single, widowed and divorced than among the married.

Table 2.1 Mortality, all causes: ratio of mortality rate of the unmarried/mortality rate of the married; whites aged 25–64, US

Marital status	Sex	Ratio
Single	Male	1.96
	Female	1.68
Widowed	Male	2.64
	Female	1.77
Divorced	Male	3.39
	Female	1.95

Source: Gove 1979. Adapted

There is also an accumulating body of research which suggests that a lack of social support or close social and emotional ties increases vulnerability to disease and the risk of death. An early study was reported by Berkman and Syme (1979), who followed a random sample of 5000 adults over a nine-year period. At the start of the study a social network index was calculated for each subject based on marital status, contacts with friends and relatives, and membership of religious or other social organizations. Over the nine-year period, mortality rates among those with a low network score were two to three times as high as those with more extensive social contacts. This kind of work completely overturns the doctrine of specific aetiology which is central to the germ theory of disease. Here, broad, non-specific social and psychological processes are seen to be associated with a variety of health outcomes.

The concept of psychosomatic illness

These four theories of the causes of disease have been presented in more or less chronological order. From the brief descriptions offered, it can be seen that the role ascribed to social and psychological factors increases immeasurably in the transition from the germ theory to the theory of general susceptibility. This should not be taken to mean that the part played by these influences has been realized only in modern times. Many cultures have viewed disease in social terms, as the outcome of disordered social relationships. In the context of modern medical history, however, the idea that disease can be ascribed to psychological causes is most commonly associated with the work of Freud. The Freudian view, which emerged at approximately the same time as the germ theory, explained conditions such as gastric ulcers and asthma in terms of the physical response to unresolved psychological conflict. The term 'psychosomatic disease' has often been used to refer to these diseases. In the 1930s the concept was revived by Jelliffe and taken to mean the complete interrelationship between functions of the mind and the body, between which no real separation could be made (Krasner 1978). This was the forerunner of the holistic approach to health subsequently adopted by Selye (1956).

Although the contemporary approach to social and psychological factors in illness has little to do with Freud, the Freudian legacy has been an unfortunate one, largely because of the association of psychosomatic illness with psychoanalytic concepts. As Fitzpatrick (1986b) notes, psychosomatic illness is often taken to mean illness that is 'imaginary' or 'not really there'. In addition, there is a lingering impression that while some diseases may be psychological in origin, most are not. The current view is that social and psychological factors are causally implicated in *all* disorders, although the mechanisms by means of which they affect health outcomes are variable.

Social factors and illness

The link between social factors and illness is evident in the association between at-risk behaviours such as smoking and lung cancer. Broad social factors such as socioeconomic status are also related to the risk of illness and death (see Chapter 3). Associations have also been observed between ethnicity, religion, sex and health outcomes. One of the more striking observations with respect to ethnicity and health concerns the differences in mortality from cerebrovascular and cardiovascular disease between the Japanese and Japanese who are resident in the US. The latter have rates which are twice as high as those of the former. The effects of migration and acculturation into the American way of life are considered to be the significant factors influencing the higher rates among expatriate Japanese.

Because religion may prescribe or proscribe patterns of behaviour it can be an important factor with respect to observed rates of individual disease or classes of disease. Mormons and Seventh Day Adventists, for example, have very low rates of all forms of cancer and this has been ascribed to their abstinence from alcohol, tobacco and caffeine.

Sex is both a biological and a social factor, and this sometimes complicates identification of the processes which account for differences in patterns of health between men and women. Simply put, men have higher rates of death while women have higher rates of illness. Some of these differences are linked to biology. For example, prior to menopause women are hormonally protected against coronary heart disease. However, the social role of women exerts an effect and can increase the risk of disease for some. Clerical workers with children, who face the combined stresses of a low status job, role expectations at work which foster submissiveness and suppression of anger, and heavy domestic duties have an increased probability of heart disease (Haynes and Feinleb 1980).

Early research on social factors and illness focused on issues such as bereavement, mobility and migration, role conflicts at work, and cultural change. More recent work has used a broader and more systematic approach, and attempts to assess the effect of life events on illness. These events generally involve some kind of loss or difficulty or are otherwise stressful. Standardized scales for measuring the frequency and severity of such life events have been developed and provide the foundation for this area of epidemiological enquiry. Using standardized scales and more innovative measurement techniques a number of researchers have identified links between life events and psychiatric illness, myocardial infarction, disturbances in the control of diabetes, and duodenal ulcers (Fitzpatrick 1986b).

The stress – disease model

The most important concept which underlies all attempts to understand the influence of social and psychological factors on health is that of stress. Stress, which can be defined as the adaptive response of an organism to a threatening stimulus, provides the link between the psychological and physiological processes which are implicated in the onset of disease. It goes without saying that psychological or emotional arousal is accompanied by quite obvious physiological responses.

At its simplest, the stress – disease model can be represented as follows:

Social environment/ social circumstances → Psychological/ emotional states → Physiological processes

↓

Disease/ susceptibility to disease

The concept of stress embraces the psychological – physiological component of the model. The basic argument is that aspects of the social environment which involve a degree of threat lead to psychological stress and a physical response in the form of changes in hormone levels and suppression of the immune system. The long-term effects of the hypersecretion of cortisol and epinephrine and the effects of stress on the autonomic nervous system have been suggested as major causes of damage to the body and its component systems. Cortisol affects the metabolism of carbohydrates, protein, and lipids. It increases gluconeogenesis in the liver, stimulates catabolic actions on muscle and lymphoid, adipose and connective tissue, and has an immunosuppressive effect (Troxler 1986). Severe mental and physical stress has been shown to increase levels of adrenocorticotrophic hormone, a precursor of cortisol, by a factor of 20. However, when stress is chronic rather than acute large individual variations in physiological response have been observed.

Selye, who did most of the initial work on stress and its consequences, called this hormonal response to stress the 'general adaptation syndrome' (Selye 1956). These changes damage body tissues directly or make the body more susceptible to noxious agents such as bacteria or viruses. It is also the case that psychological stress can lead to an increased exposure to noxious agents. For example, at times of stress people may smoke or drink more, or pay less attention to oral hygiene (Fleck-Kandath *et al.* 1988) and it is this combination of increased exposure and increased susceptibility which makes the individual disease-prone. Consequently, we can expand the basic stress–disease model in the following way.

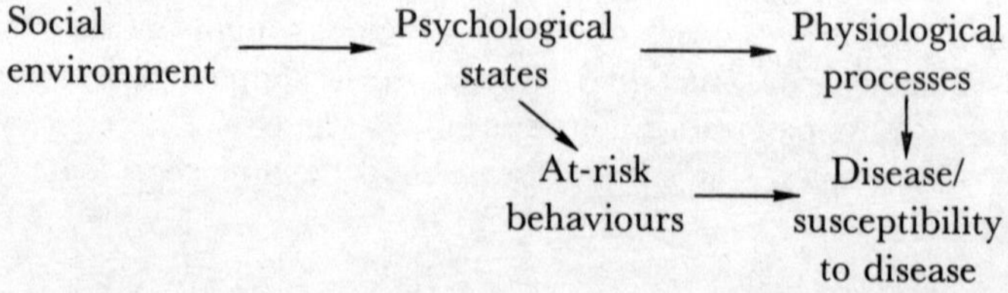

Experimental work with both animals and humans and recent research evidence concerning the health impact of stressful life events have demonstrated that the basic models presented above need to be modified to take account of additional factors. The current view is that *precipitating factors* in the form of stressors interact with *mediating factors* to affect health outcomes. These mediating factors may be personal or social, and either increase or decrease an individual's vulnerability to disease in the face of stress.

One important mediating factor having an influence on the impact of a potentially stressful event is the extent to which the individual perceives that event as threatening. Laboratory experiments have shown that the emotional and physiological arousal which accompanies a set of visually disturbing images can be modified by manipulating an individual's perception of those images (Lazarus 1966). Another factor having an important mediating effect is the individual's ability to cope with the stressor. This may involve the psychological capacity to neutralize the threat involved or the capacity to adapt to life change. In turn, these are related to an individual's personality traits and the habitual ways in which the individual responds to life events. The association between Type A behaviour — characterized by competitiveness, aggressiveness, impatience and constant striving for achievement — and heart disease is well known (Friedman and Rosenman 1974). It is not difficult to see that this association can be understood as the outcome of the ways in which Type A personalities respond psychologically and physiologically to daily life. For example, when faced with stressful situations, Type A personalities respond by higher than average secretions of cortisol and catecholamines. Consequently, cholesterol levels have been found to be higher in Type A than Type B personalities (Troxler 1986), which, in turn, is a risk factor for CHD.

While personality factors were prominent in research undertaken during the 1950s and 1960s, current efforts have been directed at clarifying the influence of social support on health. The most systematic evidence of the role of social support in the onset of specific disorders is to be found in research on depression. Among women experiencing stressful life events or long-term life difficulties, close and confiding social relationships had a protective effect, modifying the impact of such problems by preventing the demoralization and low self-esteem which preceded the onset of clinical depression (Brown and Harris 1978). The main theoretical issue in this major area of research has been whether social contacts and social ties have an independent effect on health or whether they have a buffering effect, modifying the impact of stressful life events. Because the measurement of the severity of life events, the nature and quality of social support, and health outcomes is methodologically complex, this problem has not been satisfactorily resolved.

Psychophysiological processes and oral disease

In epidemiological research in general, most studies have attempted to document the link between social–environmental stressors and health outcomes. The frequency and severity of life change events and their associations with acute or chronic health conditions have been investigated. Researchers have focused on the extremes of the stress–disease model outlined above and neglected the intervening psychological and physiological processes. In dentistry, however, the emphasis has been somewhat different, with more effort devoted to exploring the links between emotional states, physiological changes and oral disease. Here, case studies and experimental work have been more common than large scale, well-designed epidemiological studies. Nevertheless, the accumulated research evidence strongly suggests that changes in oral and systemic physiology, induced by psychological states, play an important role in the majority of oral disorders (Rugh *et al.* 1984). This is the case with respect to acute and chronic infections of both hard and soft tissues, functional disorders of the masticatory system, parafunctional behaviours and chronic orofacial pain conditions.

Stress and dental caries

Studies designed to assess the relationships between stress, personality, and dental caries have tended to be poorly designed and little confidence can be placed in their findings. For example, a number of studies have applied anxiety or personality inventories to groups of individuals and examined the associations between scores on these inventories and DMFTs. The majority of these have shown negative results. However, as Sutton (1966) argues, the anxiety and personality inventories used assess *current* psychological functioning, while the DMFT index (assuming it is an adequate measure of caries activity, which it is not) measures *past* experience of decay. Because of their design, such studies cannot hope to establish a temporal, and therefore causal, relationship between psychological factors and oral health outcomes.

The best evidence for the causal role played by stress in dental caries comes from experimental studies using animals. Research by Steinman (1960), Steinman *et al.* (1961), Sharpenak *et al.* (1963) and Borysenko *et al.* (1980) has shown that the incidence and severity of dental caries is two to three times higher in rats subject to a variety of environmental stressors when compared with non-stressed controls. Sharpenak's study is particularly useful in terms of the identification of causal pathways in that it examined the relationships between stress, diet and dental caries. There were no differences in caries activity between experimental (stressed) and control (non-stressed) groups when both were fed a non-cariogenic diet; differences emerged only when the rats were fed a cariogenic diet. This suggests that stress may only be important under certain dietary conditions.

Of the few clinical studies of stress and dental caries, the most extensive has been reported by Sutton (1965). He studied 678 patients attending a private dental practice and found 163 with acute, rapidly progressing caries lesions. A history of severe stress experiences over the previous 12 months was obtained from each subject and, in the case of those with acute caries, compared with the observer's estimate of the age of the lesions. Of the 163 patients with acute caries 159 or 97.5% reported recent mental stress. Only 2.1% of those without acute caries reported similar levels of stress.

The data also suggest a close relationship between the time of commencement of stress and the onset of acute caries.

The only epidemiological study of stress and caries examined the physical, medical and psychosocial correlates of root caries among the elderly. Using multivariate statistical techniques, Beck *et al.* (1986) were able to show that negative life events were positively associated with root decay, and the amount of participation in social activities was negatively associated with the presence of decay. Among women, negative life events made the largest single contribution to the explanation of variations in root caries.

The confidence that can be placed on the stress–caries link is increased if it can be shown that it is biologically plausible. In this case, salivary activity has been proposed as the physiological mechanism which connects the two. Saliva is believed to have a direct anti-microbial effect, reduce the adherence of bacteria to teeth and play an important role in the remineralization of surfaces subject to early decay. Evidence supporting the mediating rôle of saliva comes from clinical observation and experimental studies. For example, it has often been observed that caries becomes rampant following the onset of xerostomia. Here the salivary flow rate is severely diminished due to drugs, radiotherapy, disease, or surgical removal of the salivary glands.

Salivary flow rates are also affected by emotional stress as a result of the influence of the endocrine system on the salivary glands. Sutton (1966) states that this may also be related to personality and individual responses to stress, so that stress may increase or decrease saliva volume. The anti-bacterial activity of saliva may also be reduced by stress. Emotional stress and clinical conditions such as depression result in a suppression of the immune system which lowers the secretory IgA content of saliva.

Of course, it is also possible that behavioural as well as physiological factors are implicated in the stress–caries link. Although no studies have examined the impact of stress on health-related behaviours, it is entirely plausible that during periods of social and emotional upheaval changes in diet and oral hygiene occur which alter the oral environment and increase an individual's susceptibility to oral disease.

Soft tissue disorders

The most common soft tissue disorders observed in dental practice are periodontal disease, acute necrotizing ulcerative gingivitis (ANUG), apthous ulcers, and recurrent herpes labialis (RHL). Although the literature is not systematic, clinical observations, cross-sectional studies, and experimental work with animals all suggest that stress plays an aetiological role.

The clinical and cross-sectional studies of psychological states and periodontal disease tend to be small in scale and use standardized personality inventories to assess anxiety and other emotional characteristics of individuals with and without the disease. While most report some relationship between the two, some have produced negative findings. However, the results of studies do tend to be more consistent in suggesting that stress is a causal factor when populations exposed to naturally occurring stressful events have been studied.

Again, the plausibility of the link between stress and periodontal disease depends upon the identification of potential biological mechanisms which connect the two. A number of such physiological pathways have been suggested. Stress-induced changes in salivary flow, leading to excess build-up of calculus (in the case of increased flow) and plaque (where the flow decreases) are believed by Gupta (1966) to be the mechanism responsible. Others have suggested the direct effect of changing levels of corticosteriods on the gingival and periodontal tissues, the metabolic effects of changes in vascularization, or a generalized reduction in tissue resistance to bacterial toxins. Similar mechanisms have been suggested to account for the increased incidence of ANUG among those under some form of environmental stress.

Temporomandibular joint disorders

The term 'temporomandibular joint disorders' includes a variety of ill-defined clinical conditions characterized by pain, limitations in mandibular movement, joint sounds, and muscle tenderness. Although precise estimates of prevalence are unavailable, signs and symptoms of these conditions are relatively common in the general population. For example, a recent Canadian study found that forty-eight per cent of a sample of the general population reported one or more symptoms of TMJ syndrome and between four and ten per cent of these would probably be candidates for treatment (Locker and Slade 1988). These signs and symptoms are believed to be the product of a number of factors, including lack of posterior support, occlusal disharmony, parafunctional behaviours such as clenching and grinding, and muscle hyperactivity. In the case of the last two, stress has been proposed as an important precipitating factor.

Many experimental and clinical studies, often comparing TMJ patients with non-patient controls, have provided evidence of a correlation between stress, muscle hyperactivity, and TMJ problems. Both Kydd (1959) and Thomas *et al.* (1973) found an increase in the activity levels of muscles of the masticatory system among TMJ patients who were exposed to stressful situations, while only mimimal muscle activity was observed among the controls. Naturally occurring stressful events were shown by Rugh and Solberg (1974) to result in increased nocturnal masseter muscle activity, while Clark *et al.* (1981) demonstrated that this was related to the symptoms of TMJ dysfunction.

From an epidemiological perspective, a number of studies have investigated the relationship between stressful life events and temporomandibular joint problems. A cross-sectional study found statistically significant relationships between frequent stress, parafunctional behaviours, and the symptoms of TMJ disorders (Locker and Slade 1988). Those reporting both stress and parafunctional behaviours were almost nine times as likely to experience symptoms as those without these risk factors (Table 2.2.).

Table 2.2 Percentage reporting TMJ symptoms by presence of risk factors

Risk factor	%	Odds ratio
Stress and parafunctional behaviours	80.0	8.8
Parafunctional behaviours alone	56.9	3.5
Stress alone	47.5	2.4
Neither risk factor	31.2	1.0

Source: Compiled from data in Locker and Slade (1988)

A number of retrospective studies have also examined the association between stressful life events and temporomandibular problems. Using a standardized measure of stressful life changes, Stein *et al.* (1982) found significantly higher scores among a group of TMJ patients undergoing therapy when compared with a control group matched for age and sex. Speculand *et al.* (1984) compared the frequency of stressful life events among 85 TMJ patients and 85 non-TMJ controls. For the TMJ patients the reference period was the six months prior to the onset of pain, while for the controls it was the six months prior to the research interview. The data from the study are presented in Table 2.3.

Table 2.3 Frequency of stressful life events among TMJ cases and non-TMJ controls

No. of events	TMJ cases	Non-TMJ controls
None	23	43
One	34	33
Two	14	9
Three or more	14	0
Total	85	85

$p < 0.001$
Source: Speculand *et al.* 1984

As the table shows, there were significant differences in the occurrence of life events between the two groups. The odds ratio was 2.5, indicating that those experiencing such events were more than twice as likely to acquire TMJ dysfunction than those not. There was also evidence of a dose response relationship whereby the odds ratio increased along with increasing exposure to stressful life events. The odds ratio was 1.9 for one event but rose to 5.8 for two or more. More large-scale studies of this kind are required in order to confirm these estimates of risk and to assess the relative contribution of stress and occlusal factors to the likelihood of onset of the disorder.

The clinical significance of stress

It should be obvious from the above discussion that stress does not *cause* disease. Rather, stress is part of a complex process which, under certain circumstances, increases susceptibility to disease. The link between stress and disease is probably more direct for psychological than physical disorders, but even here its effects are moderated by mediating factors. Clarifying the role of stress in disease is important in order to better appreciate the value of stress management in treating patients with various disorders. However, it should be realized that stress reduction will not necessarily resolve existing conditions simply because other factors are involved which might need to be addressed in therapeutic endeavours. The data presented by Speculand *et al.* (1984) suggest that approximately 42 per cent of cases of TMJ disorder can be attributed to stressful life events. In those individuals where stress is not causally implicated, therapies other than those directed at stress are more appropriate.

As Krasner (1978) noted in his paper on the clinical implications of stress, recognition of the aetiological role of stress in dental and oral disorders is an important consideration in treatment planning. In the case of temporomandibular disorders, such recognition may lead to the prescription of psychological or behavioural therapies such as general relaxation training, stress control and biofeedback therapy. These have been shown to be of benefit to some patients with TMJ problems.

The role of such therapies in disorders of the hard and soft oral tissues is, however, less clear cut. Dentistry has developed a set of procedures, directed at local aetiological factors, which have largely been shown to be efficacious. Since these diseases are multifactorial, such approaches should not be abandoned in favour of treatments designed to modify stress. Patients with periodontal disease should be brought to optimal levels of oral hygiene and taught how to maintain those levels through a home care programme, irrespective of the extent to which stress is related to their problem.

However, as Krasner also notes, patients whose oral health status changes under conditions of stress can be difficult and frustrating to treat, for a deterioration in oral health may continue in spite of dental treatment, under the influence of factors which lie outside the control of the practitioner. There are a number of reports of severe emotional stress resulting in sudden periodontal breakdown even when oral hygiene standards have not deteriorated (Marco 1976). An understanding of the effects of stress can help the practitioner develop a more holistic view of the patient and promotes a practitioner–patient relationship in which conflict is minimized. This relationship is enhanced when it is realized that health is subject to influences in the social environment and need not be indicative of lapses on the part of the patient or a lack of clinical skill on the practitioner's part. Where stress has been judged to be a significant causal factor in a patient's oral health problems, Krasner suggests that treatment planning should take this into account. Such patients should be treated conservatively until they have reached a point where treatment can proceed with the maximum likelihood of a satisfactory outcome.

3

Inequalities in health and dental health

A continuing decline in death rates and increases in life expectancy demonstrate that the health of people living in the industrialized nations has improved dramatically over the course of the nineteenth and twentieth centuries. However, in spite of a general rise in living standards, the development of health care systems, and the availability of high technology medicine, fundamental inequalities in health persist. Some social groups within industrial societies are markedly healthier than others with lower death rates, less illness and disability, and better oral health. This chapter examines and attempts to explain such inequalities.

There are a number of reasons why inequalities in health need to be addressed. Understanding the social distribution of death and disease is an essential step in identifying the causes of ill health. For example, the observation that Seventh Day Adventists have lower than average rates of coronary heart disease and Jewish women have lower rates of cervical cancer than their non-Jewish counterparts provides important clues about the causes of these conditions. An understanding of the lifestyle and other factors responsible for disease demonstrates the many significant links between society and health and reminds us of the limited role played by formal health care systems in improving the health of populations.

Another reason is a concern for social justice. If health care is seen as a human right rather than a commodity to be bought by those who have the means to pay, inequalities in health become a moral and political issue. This is the case whether health care is publicly or privately funded. To the extent that differences in health are socially and economically determined, created by communities rather than immutable, the health of the most disadvantaged groups can be improved.

Dimensions of inequality

Socioeconomic status is the characteristic most commonly used in the analysis of social inequalities in health. All industrialized nations have some system for classifying their populations into socioeconomic strata or groups. In the UK the system most frequently used is the Registrar General's classification of social class. This was originally developed for the census of 1911 and, with modifications, is the basic means of classification employed by the Government's Office of Population Censuses and Surveys (OPCS). The system is based on occupation and consists of six categories which identify segments of the population sharing broadly similar types and amounts of resources and broadly similar lifestyles. The six categories comprising the scale are listed below, along with examples of their constituent occupations.

- I Professional (doctor, dentist, lawyer)
- II Managerial and lower professional (manager, nurse, schoolteacher)
- IIIN Non-manual skilled (clerk, cashier)
- IIIM Skilled manual (carpenter, bricklayer, coal face worker)
- IV Semi-skilled manual (postman, agricultural worker)
- V Unskilled manual (porter, ticket collector, general labourer)

In the US and Canada more complex classification systems are used in which occupation, income and education are combined to produce a composite rating. In addition to composite scales, income and education are often used independently as indicators of socioeconomic status.

There are a number of variables other than socioeconomic status which are related to health and overall life chances. Regional or geographical differences occur, as do differences by age, sex, race or ethnic origin, marital status, and employment status. The significance attached to these dimensions of inequality varies according to the political culture of individual countries. In Canada, for example, provincial differences in health are emphasized, while in the US more emphasis is placed on differences between the white and non-white segments of the population. In this chapter, however, only socioeconomic differences in health will be examined. Arguably, such differences are the most important and often underlie, though do not totally explain, racial and geographic differences in health. In both the US and the UK, for example, there is a close association between race or ethnic origin and socioeconomic status.

Socioeconomic differences in mortality and morbidity

Table 3.1 shows UK data relating to social class and mortality. There are clear and consistent social class gradients for males and females with respect to stillbirth rates, infant mortality rates, and standardized mortality ratios. Standardized mortality ratios are obtained by means of a statistical procedure in which death rates

Table 3.1 Social class and death from all causes: UK 1970–2

Social class	Stillbirth rate		Infant mortality rate		SMR* 1–14	SMR* 15–64
	M	F	M	F		
Professional	9	9	14	10	74	77
Intermediate	10	10	15	12	79	81
Skilled non-manual	11	12	17	12	95	99
Skilled manual	12	13	19	15	98	106
Semi-skilled	13	13	22	17	112	114
Unskilled	17	18	35	27	162	137

* Males only
Source: OPCS 1978. Adapted

are adjusted to take account of the different age compositions of the social classes so they can be compared. As the table shows, the risk of dying in the first year of life is two to three times greater for children of unskilled manual workers than for children of those in professional occupations, and this increased risk persists throughout the lifespan.

Similar social class gradients have been observed for a wide range of health measures, including acute and chronic illness rates, days of restricted activity, psychiatric symptoms, high blood pressure, height, obesity, low birth weight, prematurity, ability to conceive and self-perceived health. On all measures, whether objective clinical indicators or self-reported indicators, the lower social classes are markedly disadvantaged when compared to those at the higher end of the occupational hierarchy (MacIntyre 1986). Data demonstrating these gradients have been reported extensively for the UK since the 1950s.

Socioeconomic gradients with respect to mortality and morbidity have also been reported in Canada and the US. In both countries data collected routinely by government agencies and population surveys show that those on low incomes are significantly less healthy than those on higher incomes. In Canada, the analysis of mortality data and data from the Canada Health Survey provides a wealth of evidence of the poorer health status of the lower socioeconomic groups (Manga 1987). In addition, Wilkins and Adams (1983) have used composite health indicators to show that overall life expectancy, years of life free of disability, and quality-adjusted life years are directly related to income (see Figure 3.1). Essentially the same findings have been reported by the US Department of Health, Education and Welfare with respect to the association between health and income in the US (Department of Health Education and Welfare 1979).

In the UK the recording of occupation on the death certificate means that trends in social class differences in mortality can be monitored. This is not as easy as it seems, due to changes in occupational classification and the changing age structures of the different social classes. However, analyses of the data taking account of these changes show that the gap in mortality indicators between Class I and Classes IV and V has widened rather than diminished, in spite of the provision of free health care since 1948. The gap between the rich and the poor grew particularly sharply during the economic recession of 1979 to 1983, as a result of the combined effects of poverty and unemployment.

Inequalities in oral health

In assessing the oral health status of populations, dentistry has used a relatively narrow range of measures and indicators (see Chapter 5). Moreover, two of the major measures used, edentulism rates and DMFT scores, are somewhat unsatisfactory in that they reflect

Figure 3.1 Health expectancy by income level by age. Canada 1978

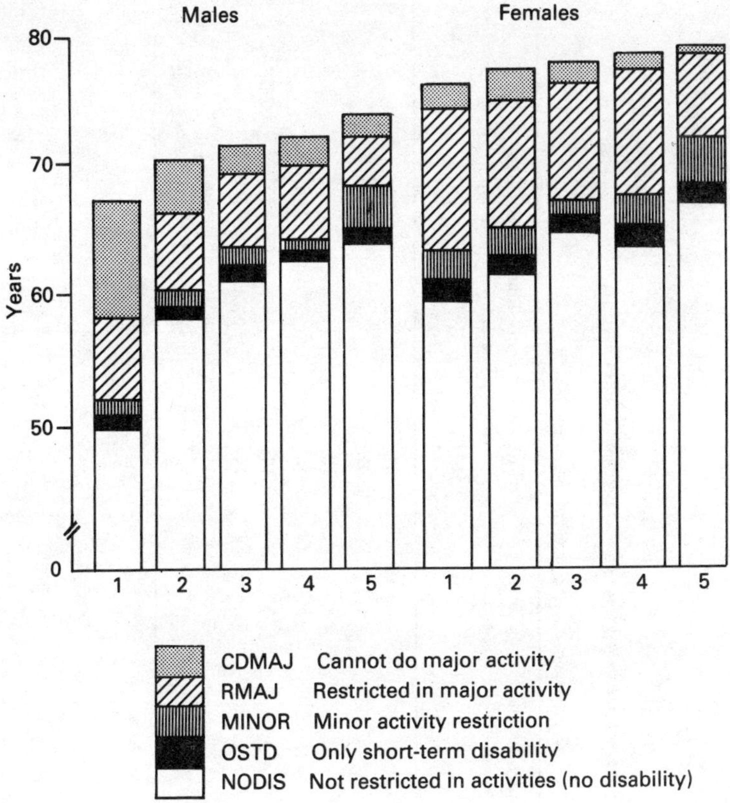

Notes: Income levels are as follows:

1. Lowest quintile
2. Second quintile
3. Third quintile
4. Fourth quintile
5. Highest quintile

Source: Wilkins and Adams 1983

disease experience *and* past experience of treatment. Nevertheless, in the majority of studies reported to date, the clinical indices used show a clear-cut and consistent association between socioeconomic status, however measured.

Table 3.2 *Total tooth loss: percentage of adults with no natural teeth by age and socioeconomic status UK, 1983*

Age (years)	Percentage with no natural teeth								
	Professional	Employers and managers	Intermediate non-manual	Junior non-manual	Skilled manual and own account non-professional	Semi-skilled manual and personal service	Unskilled manual	All non-manual	All manual
16–24	nil	nil	nil	*	*	nil	1	*	*
25–34	nil	2	1	1	2	3	5	1	3
35–44	2	4	7	4	12	14	23	4	13
45–54	6	11	15	16	28	35	38	12	31
55–64	15	28	26	36	48	58	59	28	53
65–74	28	45	42	60	74	77	75	48	75
75 and over	**	73	74	77	84	89	88	73	87
All aged 16 and over	8	19	16	20	28	36	44	18	32

* Less than one per cent
** Base number too small to allow percentaging
Source: OPCS 1986

The relationship between socioeconomic status and caries experience has been investigated by numerous studies in the UK, US, Scandinavia, and Australasia. In a review of the studies published between 1941 and 1978, Carmichael *et al.* (1980) found that thirty-three reported a higher caries experience in the lower social classes, five reported no differences and two reported a reduced caries experience in the lower social classes. In those studies in which no differences were found, tooth loss was greater in the lower social classes, reflecting a more frequent resort to extraction rather than restoration.

Table 3.2 shows the relationship between age, socioeconomic status and tooth loss in the UK (OPCS 1986). For this analysis an expanded version of the Registrar General's classification was used. Rates of tooth loss ranged from a low of 8 per cent among professionals to a high of 44 per cent among those in unskilled manual occupations, a gradient evident in all age groups. The columns to the far right of the table show that people in the manual group were almost twice as likely to have lost all their teeth than those in the non-manual group except at ages 55 and over. An even greater social class gradient in edentulousness has been reported in New Zealand. Data from a WHO study found that 64 per cent of unskilled manual workers had lost all their teeth compared with none of those in professional and similar occupations (Davis 1981). In the US levels of edentulism are directly related to both income and education, with rates 3 to 5 times as high in the lowest income and educational groups as in the highest (US Department of Health Education and Welfare 1979). These relationships were also observed in recent national surveys of employed and older adults (Meskin *et al.* 1988). Other studies have found that comparable social class differences exist in the presence of untreated decay, the presence of conditions needing immediate treatment, periodontal health, and oral hygiene status (Nikias *et al.* 1975). In all cases, those on low incomes or with the lowest levels of education have the worst oral health experience (see Table 3.3).

Similar social class differences in oral health have been found in children. Infante and Owen (1975) used data from a dental health survey of children in the US and found that children of low socioeconomic status had higher mean deft and defs scores at all ages than children of higher socioeconomic status. The former experienced decay at an earlier age, had a greater rate of attack and were less likely to be caries free. National oral health surveys in the UK (Todd and Dodd 1985) and local surveys in the US

Table 3.3 Oral health status in relation to socioeconomic status: urban adults in the USA

	Socioeconomic status		
	Low	Medium	High
Percentage with:			
Six or more missing teeth	60	48	35
Medium or high periodontal disease	58	53	41
OHI-S* greater than 2.0	49	37	42
Decayed teeth ratio greater than 0%**	55	44	39
Filled teeth ratio less than 100%***	62	49	42

* Simplified oral hygiene index
** Decayed teeth as proportion of teeth present
*** Filled teeth as proportion of teeth attacked by decay
Source: Nikias *et al.* 1977

(Szwejda 1960; Szwejda 1962) and Scandinavia (Hausen *et al.* 1981) have reported the same trends.

The examination of trends in oral health status by social class requires repeated cross-sectional surveys on the same populations using the same methods and procedures. Adult oral health surveys conducted in the UK in 1968, 1978 and 1983 suggest that rates of edentulism are falling (from 37% in 1968 to 25% in 1983) and that between 1968 and 1978 they fell more steeply in the lower classes. A failure to use age-standardized rates means that these conclusions are difficult to assess.

Explaining socioeconomic differences in health

The most systematic attempt to explain socioeconomic differences in health was made by the Working Group on Inequalities in Health appointed by the UK Government in 1977. This Working Group, which reported in 1980, reviewed data concerning health inequalities in Britain and examined a number of competing explanations (Townsend and Davidson 1982). Although their report did not cover oral health and dental health services the following theories and approaches are equally applicable to dental conditions.

The artefact explanation

This theory does not explain inequalities in health but denies their existence. It tends to be favoured by statisticians and social scientists who are sceptical of routinely collected data. They would argue that the differences revealed by the data presented in Tables 3.1 to 3.3 are not real but artificial, the product of our attempts to measure complex entities with inadequate measurement tools. Health is multidimensional (see Chapter 4) and we must often use indicators which are far from satisfactory. Moreover, they claim that age differences among the socioeconomic groups, changes in the classification of occupations over time, and historical changes in the occupational structure of modern societies make it virtually impossible to assess trends in inequalities in health. These doubts concerning the data on socioeconomic differences in health are not entirely without merit. Nevertheless, the evidence concerning health inequalities is overwhelming. Systematic gradients exist between those at the top and bottom of the socioeconomic scale whether we use objective or subjective indicators of health, and whether socioeconomic status is measured by occupation, education, or income.

The theory of natural and social selection

The data in Tables 3.1 to 3.3 demonstrate the existence of an *association* between socioeconomic status and health but say nothing about the direction of the causal link. While it is easy to appreciate that socioeconomic status influences health, it is also possible that health has an influence on socioeconomic status. The theory of natural and social selection subscribes to this latter point of view. This theory claims that inequalities in health are created and maintained by a process of social mobility whereby healthy individuals move up the social hierarchy while the less healthy move down. Health is seen as a prerequisite for economic success and determines an individual's place in the class structure. The widening of socioeconomic differences in health is explained by the fact that modern societies are more open and fluid than they were and present greater opportunities for upward mobility to the fit and able. Consequently, over time, the upper socioeconomic groups have become increasingly healthy relative to those at the bottom of the social hierarchy.

This theory is supported by those few studies which have examined the relationship between health and social mobility. These studies confirm that chronic conditions such as schizophrenia and chronic bronchitis lead to a downward occupational drift, often ending in low paid, unskilled manual labour or unemployment. More systematic studies by Illsley (1980) have demonstrated a link between the health status of women and social mobility at marriage. A study published in 1955 and repeated in 1980 revealed that the healthiest women were more likely to be upwardly mobile at marriage, marrying men from a socio-economic group higher than their own, while less healthy women were more likely to be downwardly mobile. This concentration of less healthy women in the lowest social classes partially explains the higher perinatal mortality rate among this group.

There is also evidence to suggest a link between oral health status and social mobility. A substantial literature has indicated that dental conditions significantly affect facial attractiveness and can have an important influence on an individual's chances in life, particularly with respect to educational and occupational success. This research is reviewed in Chapter 6.

Although these studies demonstrate that health *can* have an effect on socioeconomic status the magnitude of that effect is questionable. After reviewing all the arguments and major studies of the determinants of social mobility, Blane (1985) concluded that the influence of health was small.

The materialist explanation

The remaining explanations considered by the Working Group on Inequalities in Health can be called social causation theories. Here, socioeconomic status is accorded a causal role and seen to be a major determinant of health. The materialist explanation reviewed here, and the cultural explanation reviewed below, claim that socioeconomic status has a significant influence on exposure to health hazards and resistance to disease. The two explanations, however, differ in terms of the mechanisms that are believed to be responsible for the link between the two.

Materialist explanations suggest that inequalities in health have their origins in material deprivation. Simply put, the lower socio-economic groups lack adequate resources to maintain their physical and psychological health and to protect themselves from hazardous natural or artificial environments (Hart 1985). Although living standards have risen remarkably and consistently over the course of the twentieth century, fundamental inequalities persist in the material circumstances and conditions of life. Many people, for example, continue to live in, or on the margins of, poverty, unable to provide themselves or their families with the basic amenities of daily living.

Most of the evidence linking material deprivation and poor health has focused on differences in income and wealth, working conditions, and the quality of housing and the domestic environment. The lower socioeconomic groups are often severely disadvantaged in terms of all three. The relationship between such deprivation and health has been demonstrated in numerous studies. Data from the UK, for example, show that a close association exists between income and the risk of dying. Similarly, evidence of the impact of working conditions on health abounds and a wide range of diseases have been shown to be associated with physical and chemical hazards at work. Such hazards are obviously more common in manual occupations, which are physically more arduous and in which exposure to dust, chemicals and noise is much more likely. The hazards involved in manual occupations are also reflected in statistics concerning deaths due to accidents at work. Again, data from the UK demonstrate that men in unskilled manual occupations are more than ten times as likely to die from such accidents as their professional counterparts. Other differences in working conditions have a less direct, although significant, effect on health and exert their influence through psychosocial mechanisms such as stress. A number of Swedish studies have shown that lack of security of tenure, low job satisfaction, machine-paced work, monotonous and repetitive tasks, a lack of autonomy and close supervision lead to an increased output of stress hormones and have been linked to an increased risk of heart disease (Blane 1985).

Socioeconomic differences in the health of children have been shown to result from poor quality housing and hazardous domestic environments. Overcrowding, damp conditions and inadequate heating all have an effect on health and are associated with increased rates of death from respiratory illness and accidents in the home. Children drawn from the lower social classes are more at risk from traffic accidents and lead pollution, and are more likely to live in areas with higher than average levels of pollution by industrial waste such as sulphur dioxide and particulate matter in the form of smoke.

It is clear that no single factor from among those listed above can adequately explain socioeconomic differences in health. It is much more likely that such factors interact to produce these differences. One of the few studies to examine a combination of factors attempted to explain the higher rates of depressive illness in working-class women (Brown and Harris 1979). Working-class women were more likely than middle-class women to encounter stressful life events which involved a long-term loss or threatened self-esteem. These usually took the form of problems with housing, financial affairs, and family crises. Working-class women were also found to be more vulnerable to these psychological stressors because they lacked the personal and social resources which enabled middle-class women to cope with such stress. Studies such as this demonstrate quite clearly that health is socially and environmentally determined.

As yet there is very little comparable evidence to indicate a link between the material conditions of life and oral health. Such evidence, however, is beginning to appear in the scientific literature. This largely concerns the association between stress and vulnerability to oral conditions and was reviewed in Chapter 2. A study which has investigated the relationship between occupational status, the work environment, and oral disorders has recently been reported from Sweden. Enbom *et al.* (1986) studied the degree of occlusal wear and frequency of clinical signs of temporomandibular dysfunction in two groups of miners: one had been working in mines for 5 to 7 years and the other for 10 years or more. They were compared with two matched groups of white collar workers. Both groups of miners had significantly higher degrees of occlusal wear than their respective white collar controls, and the older miners had a greater frequency of signs of temporomandibular disorders. The most probable reason for this was differences in the working environments of the miners and white collar controls, particularly atmospheric pollution with abrasive particles and hyperactivity in the masticatory muscles due to work-induced stress. Similar observations have been made with respect to workers in the iron industry. In Sweden, workers, with severe occlusal wear are entitled to compensation under the Industrial Injuries Insurance Act.

Cultural or behavioural theories

Cultural or behavioural theories attempt to explain inequalities in health in terms of social class differences in knowledge, attitudes and behaviours. People in the lower socioeconomic groups are believed to be less healthy because they more frequently consume health-damaging substances such as tobacco and alcohol, eat diets which are high in fats and sugars and low in fibres, are less likely to include exercise in their leisure activities and make less use of preventive health services such as dental visits, immunization and antenatal care.

This explanation is valid to the extent that there are class differences in lifestyle and consumption patterns, and these have been implicated in the onset of major killers such as heart disease and cancer, and non-fatal conditions such as dental decay. The problem with this explanation is that it has an overly simplistic view of behaviours such as smoking, alcohol use and diet: they are seen as matters of individual choice which can be modified by health education. Blane (1985) has argued that the reasons for these behaviours are more complex and are to be found in the material conditions of life of the lower socioeconomic groups. In a sense, behavioural theories are really part and parcel of materialist explanations of health inequalities.

Blane supports his argument by examining the physiological and psychological properties of nicotine. Nicotine is a mood-altering drug which allays fatigue and enhances performance during monotonous tasks. The attraction of nicotine for those whose work involves repetitive and routine activities, primarily clerical, skilled, and unskilled manual labour, seems obvious. It is interesting to note that the increase in smoking among women has paralleled their increased participation in the work force, a participation which commits many women to such routine, repetitive labour.

Because cultural/behavioural theories tend to be favoured by health care professionals and health educators, evidence concerning socioeconomic differences in knowledge, attitudes, and behaviours — and their relationship to dental disease — is relatively plentiful. Persons from the upper socioeconomic groups tend to be more knowledgeable about dental disorders and their causes. This is a function of higher educational levels and a greater interest in the maintenance of health. Beal (1983) found that 83 per cent of mothers from social class I knew of the importance of frequency of sugar consumption in the onset of dental caries compared to 59 per cent of mothers from social classes IV and V. These differences in knowledge are reflected in behaviours which have a bearing on oral health. The more cariogenic diets and poorer oral hygiene of children from the lower classes are the product of the kind of child care practices indicated in Table 3.4.

Table 3.4 Percentage of 5-year-old children exhibiting various patterns of behaviour related to dental health according to social class

Social class	Child brushes at least once per day	Child was given sugared dummy	More than 25p spent on sweets per week
I and II	92	17	2
III	74	29	15
IV and V	64	30	13

Source: Beal and Dickson 1974

An impression of the different attitudes and behaviours of adults towards dental health can be obtained from the data presented in Table 3.5. In dental health surveys of adults conducted in the late 1960s to the late 1970s, fewer people in social class I expressed concern at the thought of wearing dentures, more working-class than middle-class mothers preferred extraction rather than restoration of decayed teeth in five-year-old children, and only 28 per cent of classes IV and V attended for a regular dental check-up compared to 56 per cent of those in classes I and II. However, there is reason to believe that these differences in attitude and behaviour are narrowing over time.

In an analysis of barriers to preventive dentistry, Blaikie (1979) has shown how these different dental attitudes and behaviours are the product of broader cultural differences between individuals drawn from the upper and lower socioeconomic groups. The lower socioeconomic groups tend to be concerned with the present rather than the future and, because they see the future as too unpredictable to warrant long-term planning, are reluctant to undertake actions whose benefits are long-term and uncertain. Fatalism also tends to be a cultural characteristic of these lower socioeconomic groups. Life is seen as a series of events which affect the quality of their lives but over which they have little or no control. Consequently, health is believed to be a matter of luck or heredity and not something which can be influenced greatly by individual action. The loss of teeth is associated with the aging process; it is not a health issue but an inevitable part of life experience.

Again, Blane (1985) would argue that these cultural differences reflect the actual conditions of life of people in the lower classes. Their existence is characterized by insecurity, particularly with regard to employment and housing, so that long-term planning makes little real sense. In addition, people from the lower social

Table 3.5 Social class differences in behaviour and attitude in relation to dental health

Proportion of dentate adults attending for regular check-ups, 1978*	
I, II, IIIN	56%
IIIM	36%
IV and V	28%
Percentage bothered at thought of wearing dentures, 1968**	
I and II	71%
III	49%
IV	53%
V	31%
Percentage of mothers choosing extraction rather than fillings as the treatment for decayed primary teeth, 1974***	
I and II	46%
III	60%
IV and V	76%

Source: * Todd *et al.* 1982
** Gray *et al.* 1970
*** Beal and Dickson 1974

classes are likely to have the least degree of control over their own day-to-day existence. Decisions regarding education, housing and work are more than likely made by others on their behalf. Again, taking responsibility for their own health makes no sense when they are denied responsibility for much of what happens in their daily lives. It remains to be seen, of course, whether these differences in life chances and cultural orientations survive the change in the structure of societies supposed to accompany the move to a post-industrial information society.

Social class differences in access to health care

The Working Group on Inequalities in Health did not consider unequal access to health care to offer anything more than a partial explanation of social class differences in health. This is because most health care systems are curative rather than preventive in approach and have only a minor impact on the prevalence and distribution of death and disease in a population. Nevertheless, class differences in the quantity and quality of health care received need to be examined to determine how far equality of access has been achieved. Equality of access is a basic principle of the National Health Service in the UK and of comparable systems such as Canada's provincially-managed health insurance schemes whereby health services are provided free at the point of delivery.

Given that the National Health Service has been in existence for forty years it is not surprising that a great deal of data exists on inequalities in the use of health care in the UK. Data from surveys tend to show that the poor use general practitioner services more than the rich. However, studies which have taken account of *need* for medical care reveal that this gradient is reversed, with the upper socioeconomic groups consulting doctors more in relation to their level of need (Forster 1976). It has also been shown that the upper socioeconomic groups tend to be treated by doctors with more postgraduate qualifications, better equipped surgeries, and more auxiliary staff. Moreover, they are referred for specialist care more frequently than the lower socioeconomic groups (Blaxter 1984). In terms of the content of consultations, the middle class spend more time with their doctors, ask more questions, and receive more information about their condition (Cartwright and O'Brien 1976). Whether these differences result in better outcomes for middle class patients has, however, recently been questioned (Boulton *et al.* 1986).

Almost identical observations have been made with respect to the quantity and quality of dental care received. Data from the UK show that the middle class visit the dentist more regularly than the working class, they are less likely to visit only when in pain, and they take their children for dental check-ups at an earlier age. Canadian data reveal a similar pattern; white collar workers and upper income groups were more likely to have visited a dentist during the previous year (Charette 1986). A Norwegian study has recently shown that in spite of an increase in the proportion of people visiting a dentist regularly over the period 1972–1983, there was no discernible reduction in social inequalities in the use of dental services (Rise 1985). One factor which does seem to have some effect on differential patterns of use is the availability of dentists. O'Mullane and Robinson (1977) report that in a community with a favourable dentist–population ratio the use of services by the upper and lower socioeconomic groups was broadly similar, whereas in a community with a less favourable ratio the usual social class gradient was observed. Given that dentists are more numerous in areas of high social class, one way of reducing inequalities in use would be to increase the numbers of dentists practising in areas of greatest need.

There is also a great deal of evidence which demonstrates social variations in the pattern of dental treatment received. This is not confined to the UK. In New Zealand and the US the middle class also receive more restorative work and fewer extractions than the lower class. Children from the middle class are more likely to be referred for orthodontic treatment, more likely to receive treatment for minor defects in occlusion, and more likely to receive complex orthodontic therapy (Jenkins *et al.* 1984). These differences in treatment may be the product of negative attitudes on the part of the lower social classes and their preferences for treatment. They may also be influenced by dentists' attitudes towards patients of different social class backgrounds. In a study of factors related to dentists' decisions to extract rather than restore teeth, Kay and Blinkhorn (1987) report that extractions for caries were more frequent among regular than irregular attenders. Judging by the numbers of radiographs taken prior to extraction, it also appeared that the irregular attender received a less thorough type of clinical care. Since visiting patterns and social class are closely associated, this study suggests differences in the quality of dental care offered to patients of different social classes.

Reducing inequalities in health

The explanations reviewed above have different implications with respect to interventions to reduce class inequalities in health. The Working Group on Inequalities in Health tended to favour the materialist explanation and produced a series of policy recommendations designed to address broader inequalities in living conditions. These included a comprehensive anti-poverty programme, measures to discourage smoking, and improvements in housing and working conditions. They also recommended efforts to improve primary health care and efforts to stimulate the use of preventive services by those most at risk. In this regard inequalities in health are a social and political problem which can only be resolved by fundamental changes in the distribution of income and material resources. These kinds of conclusions proved somewhat unpalatable to the British government which rejected both the report and its recommendations on the grounds of their implications for public expenditure.

To the extent that knowledge, attitudes, and behaviour are implicated in socioeconomic differences in health, measures such as health education have an important role to play. How much can be achieved by these measures will depend upon the extent to which the attitudes and behaviour in question are rooted in the material circumstances of life. Similarly, improving the quality and distribution of medical and dental services is also important, but this strategy is limited in terms of how far it can narrow the gap between the classes. Services which provide treatment for already existing disease and do not address the causes of that disease are no substitute for a comprehensive strategy which seeks to promote community health.

Some interest has recently been expressed in the contribution made by public health measures such as fluoridation of the water supplies in equalizing the caries experience of children. Such interventions have the advantage that they reach the entire community and are not dependent upon favourable attitudes and dispositions among the target population. Studies conducted during the 1980s have produced inconsistent results. Surveys of children in Finland found that water fluoridation had a similar effect in all social classes (Hausen *et al.* 1981), while studies in the US and UK suggest that fluoridation has a greater preventive effect in the lower social classes, leading to the removal of class differences in caries experience (Weddell and Klein 1981, Carmichael *et al.* 1984).

Studies conducted in the north of England by the same team in 1976 and 1981 demonstrate how difficult it is to interpret the relationship between class, caries and fluoridation (Carmichael *et al.* 1984). Taken individually, both the 1976 and 1981 studies suggest that fluoridation has a greater effect on classes IV and V and narrows the gap between the upper and lower classes. For example, in 1976 there was no social class gradient in the percentage of 5-year-old children who were caries-free in the high-fluoride community but a noticeable gradient in the low-fluoride area. In 1981 there was evidence of a gradient in both communities, but that in the low-fluoride area was much steeper (see Table 3.6). However, if the results of the studies are taken together in order to reveal the rate of change over time in the highest and lowest socioeconomic groups a different picture emerges. Figure 3.2 shows quite clearly that in both low-fluoride and high-fluoride areas the improvement in the caries experience of children in classes I and II is happening more quickly than among children in

Figure 3.2 Percentage caries free, social classes I and II and IV and V by fluoridation status of the community and survey year

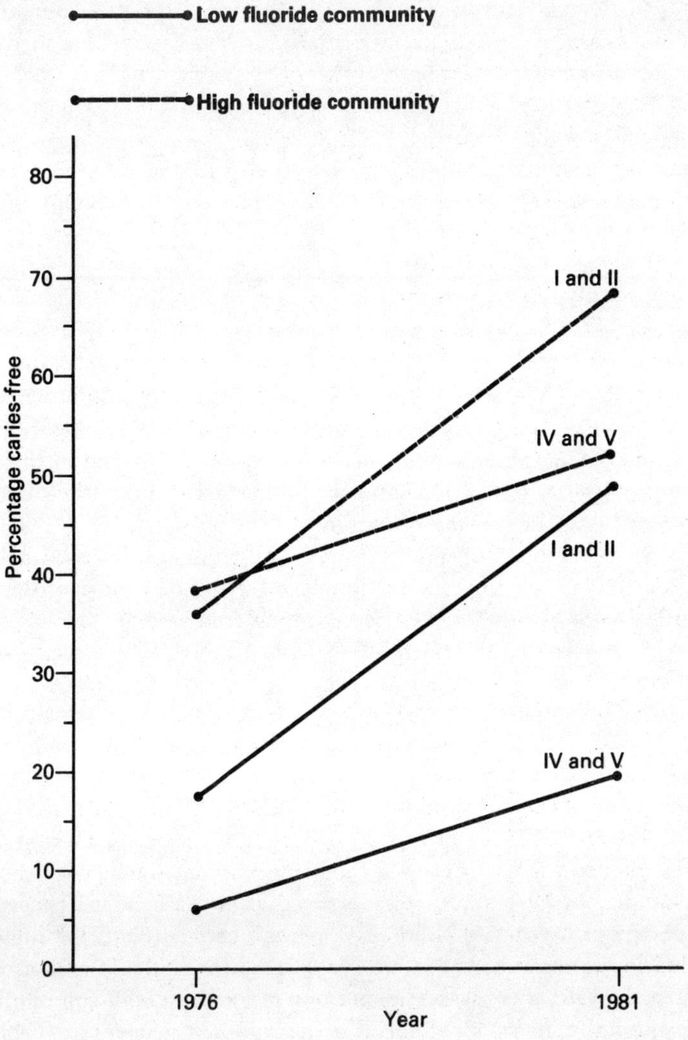

Source: Compiled from data provided by Carmichael *et al.* 1984

Table 3.6 Percentage of five-year-old children caries-free by social class, fluoridation status of the community, and year of survey

	1976		1981	
	Low fluoride	High fluoride	Low fluoride	High fluoride
I and II	17	35	48	67
III	15	33	31	52
IV and V	3	37	20	51
Difference between I and II and IV and V	+ 14	− 2	+ 28	+ 16

Source: Carmichael *et al.* 1984

classes IV and V. Note also that the rate of change as indicated by the slope of the line is similar within social classes and is independent of the fluoridation status of the community. Viewed in this way the data suggest a widening class differential in dental caries irrespective of the communities in which these children live. Where fluoridation appears to make a contribution is in reducing the extent of that differential. Should these trends continue, the residual pool of caries will be found in children who are the least likely to present for treatment. This poses a potential challenge to the dental health profession in organizing services to reach those who remain in need.

4
Aging and oral health

Children, the physically and mentally handicapped, the elderly, and the poor constitute special patient groups. These can be defined as sub-groups of the population who pose special problems either for the dental practitioner or the dental health care system as a whole. Traditionally, children have been regarded as the most important of these groups: more is known about the oral health status of, and trends in oral disease in, children than in adults, and all dental health care systems, whether publicly or privately funded, make some provision for this age group. In the UK this special provision takes the form of a school dental service and free dental treatment, while in Canada it takes the form of provincially-funded dental programmes which cover the cost of dental care for this age group.

Two major trends affecting all modern industrialized societies will mean that the significance of children as a special population group will diminish. These trends are, first, the changing pattern and distribution of dental disease in modern populations, and second, the changing age structure of those populations. Current evidence suggests that the number and proportion of children in the population will decline and the prevalence of dental decay among children will also be significantly reduced. These factors will reduce the dental treatment needs of this section of the population. Conversely, the increase in the numbers of elderly persons and the increasing tendency for elderly people to retain their own teeth means that the dental treatment needs of those over retirement age will increase dramatically. The elderly will form a major market for dental care by the year 2000 and providing for this market will, more than likely, bring about major changes in patterns of dental practice.

The aging of modern populations

Since 1900, the age-specific demographic profile of industrialized societies has been changing. The population pyramid, in which children form a broad base with a gradual tapering with age, is gradually being replaced by a structure more rectangular in shape. This means that the numbers of elderly in these populations are increasing relative to the younger age groups. This process is one which accompanies urbanization and industrialization, and may well be observed in developing countries over the next century.

The aging of modern populations is the product of low birth rates, low death rates, and the aging of large birth cohorts such as that produced by the baby-boom following World War II. If life expectancy continues to increase and the developed nations approach zero population growth then the proportion of elderly in some countries will approach 20 per cent. In developing countries, continuing high birth rates combined with a decrease in infant mortality will result in an increase in the population overall, but only moderate increases in the elderly.

In 1900, only 5 per cent of the population living in North America (Canada and the US) were over the age of 65 years. By 1980 this had risen to 9 per cent and is expected to rise to 12 per cent by 2000 and 17 per cent by 2010. By the year 2000, there will be 34 million people aged 65 years or over in North America. In the UK, 6 per cent of the population were over retirement age in 1901 and this is projected to increase to 16 per cent by 2001. Because of increasing life expectancy, the growth in the number and proportion of the 'very old', i.e. persons over the age of 75 years, will be even more dramatic. In the Province of Ontario, Canada, which has a population of just over eight million people, the numbers aged 65 to 74 years will increase by 41 per cent between 1983 and 2006, while the numbers aged 75 years and over will rise by 104 per cent. In the UK some 3 million people or 1 in 20 of the population are very old. Given the sex differences in mortality rates, a large proportion of these will be elderly women.

The change in the age structure of modern populations has a number of social and economic implications and will place significant stresses on services or institutions designed to meet the needs of the various age groups. These stresses arise because the elderly are not economically productive (owing to their mandatory exclusion from the labour force) but have high needs for medical and social care. In the UK, for example, half the non-psychiatric

NHS hospital beds are occupied by patients over the age of 65 years and the elderly are major users of general practitioner services. Some have questioned whether societies will be able to generate enough wealth to support the increasing numbers of elderly. Certainly the aged-dependency ratio, the ratio of the number of non-working elderly to active participants in the labour force, has increased. This was 29 per 100 in the UK in 1985 and will be 38 per 100 by 2025 (OPCS 1985).

The current and future elderly: aging and cohort effects

In attempting to assess differences in the health and behaviour of different age groups it is important to distinguish between aging effects and cohort effects. Aging effects are the product of growing old while cohort differences are due to the fact that people of different age groups belong to different generations which have been subject to specific social and historical experiences. These experiences, rather than aging per se, explain the observed differences between the young and the old. Age differences in attitudes and behaviours are often due to cohort effects rather than processes of biological and social aging (McPherson 1983).

For example, data which show that the elderly are less concerned with their oral health than younger age groups does not necessarily mean that people become less disposed to take care of their teeth and oral cavity as they grow old. It may be that the elderly are from a generation which has always had a negative view of dentistry while the young represent a generation which will carry more positive attitudes into old age.

Predicting the future dental care needs and demands of the elderly population means that it is important to sort out aging and cohort effects. If the differences in which we are interested are due to aging, then the current and future elderly are likely to be quite similar. Where they are due to cohort effects, then the elderly of the future will have characteristics which are different from those of the elderly of today.

Ettinger and Beck (1982) have recently described the differences in the dental health attitudes and behaviours of the 'old' elderly (those aged 75 to 80 years) and the 'new' elderly (those aged 60 to 65 years). These they attribute to the influence of different social and cultural life experiences. The old elderly were growing up at a time when dentistry was rather primitive and often performed by unlicensed practitioners. Dental treatment was considered a luxury and, for many, was sought only when in pain. The theory of focal infection was prevalent at the time (see Chapter 1) and extraction often the treatment of choice. This era in dentistry has been called the 'blood and vulcanite' period when mass extraction of teeth was the norm. Where restoration of teeth was undertaken the lack of adequate local anaesthetics and the absence of the air turbine meant that these procedures were uncomfortable if not painful. For these reasons, many of the old elderly are edentulous with a negative attitude to dentistry and the natural dentition.

Although born only 15 years later, the new elderly are likely to have had a more positive experience of dentistry. Many received free dental care while on military service during World War II and were able to take advantage of new treatment philosophies and developments in health care technology which transformed the delivery of dental care. These trends are even more likely to have affected the future elderly (those currently aged 45 to 60 years) who are not only better educated and more aware of health issues but have grown up in a period of increasing government involvement in health care provision based on the view that access to health services is as much a right as a privilege. Moreover, during their early years the stress in dentistry was on restoration and the preservation of the natural dentition while in their later years prevention has emerged as a dominant theme in health. These cohort experiences will influence both the oral health status of the future elderly and their needs and demand for dental care. In many important respects they will be different from the elderly of today.

The oral health status of the current and future elderly

In assessing the oral health status of the elderly a distinction also needs to be drawn between aging and disease. These are frequently confused, with the result that a number of stereotypes regarding the oral health of the elderly have developed and been maintained over time. Changes in the oral mucosa, salivary flow rates, oral sensory perception and changes in orofacial musculature have often been attributed to aging when they are the product of pathological processes rather than normal changes in structure and function (Baum 1981). For example, recent evidence suggests that the diminished salivary flow frequently observed in studies of the elderly is due to disease or the effect of medications and not to aging in and of itself. Similarly, high rates of tooth loss, often believed to be a natural accompaniment of growing old, are the product of pathological processes, negative attitudes to the natural dentition, and treatment philosophies which stressed extraction rather than prevention and restoration (Weintraub and Burt 1985).

The oral health status of the elderly and their trends in oral disease are difficult to characterize. Epidemiological studies of this section of the population are relatively few, they tend to be local rather than national in character, and they are usually cross-sectional. Moreover, there are differences between countries and differences within countries according to geographic location and socioeconomic status. In general, however, the elderly have high needs for dental treatment yet tend to receive less professional attention than younger age groups. Rates of edentulism are high, prosthetic replacements are often poor and the elderly have high rates of denture-related mucosal disorders. Among the dentate, coronal caries is a continuing problem, root caries a major clinical problem and periodontal disease observed around a substantial proportion of remaining teeth. These problems tend to increase with age and are particularly marked in those elderly cared for in institutions. There is also an increasing body of research to show that these problems have significant social and psychological effects on this age group and a negative impact on the quality of life (see Chapter 6).

Edentulism and tooth loss

One of the most dramatic of the age differences in oral health is in rates of edentulism and tooth loss. Both of these increase sharply with age, females having higher rates than males. The extent of the differences by age are readily apparent in Table 4.1, which shows rates for the UK for 1968, 1978 and 1983. In the early survey years more than three-quarters of those aged 65 years and above had lost all of their natural teeth.

The surveys also show that over the ten-year period between 1968 and 1978 edentulism rates fell: from 37 per cent overall in 1968 to 29 per cent overall in 1978. The rates declined for all age groups and this decline was most marked in those under the age of 65 years. The data for 1978 also show that a clear difference

Table 4.1 Trends in total tooth loss UK: percentage of adults with no natural teeth by age

	Percentage with no natural teeth		
Age (years)	1968	1978	1983
18–24	1	*	*
25–34	7	3	2
35–44	22	12	7
45–54	41	29	22
55–64	64	48	41
65–74	79	74	64
75 and over	88	87	81
All aged 16 and over	37	29	25

* Less than one per cent
Source: OPCS 1986

emerged between those over and under 65 years of age. By 1983 the overall rate had fallen to 25 per cent, with the rate for the young elderly, those aged 65 to 74 years, falling to 64 per cent. Since these data suggest that the younger age groups are keeping their teeth as they age a substantial improvement in edentulism rates should be observed in the elderly during the 1980s and continue for the remainder of the century. Using crude assumptions about the age-specific incidence of edentulism, only 20 per cent of those aged 65 to 74 and 38 per cent of those aged 75 years and over will have no natural teeth by the year 2008.

Broadly comparable data from cross-sectional studies in the US show similar trends. The oral health status of the US population is more favourable than that of the population in the UK and this is reflected in markedly lower rates of tooth loss. The overall rate of edentulism was 17 per cent in 1960–2 and 8 per cent in 1980. The figures for those aged 65 to 74 years are 49 per cent and 33 per cent respectively (Weintraub and Burt 1985). Projections indicate that this rate will have fallen to around 10 per cent by the year 2021. Consequently, by the turn of the century the age gradient in tooth loss will be far less steep and cohort differences largely eliminated.

Coronal caries

According to Baum (1981) coronal caries is often overlooked in the elderly because they are erroneously stereotyped as an almost wholly edentulous population. While information on coronal caries in this section of the population is relatively sparse, studies of selected groups of elderly have shown that it continues to be a problem. Mean numbers of decayed teeth varied from 1.5 to 6.7 in the studies reviewed by Beck (1984). In fact, national studies in the UK and regional surveys in the US provide evidence to suggest that elderly people have as high if not higher decay rates than younger adults, and much of this will be on tooth surfaces which have already been filled (Todd *et al.* 1982, Beck 1984). For example, the 1978 survey of the dental health of adults in the UK found that 62 per cent of those over the age of 55 years had active decay compared with 68 per cent of those aged 16 to 24 years. The data also show that the proportion of 16- to 24-year-olds with decay had fallen by approximately 10 per cent since an earlier survey in 1968, while the rates had remained stable for those over the age of 45. If caries prevalence rates are calculated as a percentage of teeth present and not as a percentage of persons then the differences in prevalence by age are even more striking (Chauncey 1978).

However, because these data refer to prevalence and not incidence some caution must be exercised when predicting future trends. Firstly, the elderly may have higher prevalence rates because they are less likely to receive dental treatment and not because they are at greater risk of developing dental caries. The incidence data available from the only longitudinal study of the elderly suggest that the incidence rate is high: among a sample of 447 dentate persons living independently in the community, 51 per cent acquired new coronal lesions over an 18-month period (Hand *et al.* 1988). Secondly, even if the incidence remains high in the current elderly this may be a cohort effect which will not be maintained as younger cohorts age. Nevertheless, given that more elderly people are retaining teeth, coronal decay will remain a significant public health problem even if age-specific incidence declines.

Root caries

Because root caries is related to gingival recession, it tends to be a problem of the elderly. While it does occur in young adults rates increase systematically and dramatically with age. National data on root caries were collected in two surveys recently completed in the US (US Department of Health and Human Services 1987). They show that 21 per cent of people of working age had root decay, with a mean of 0.76 decayed or filled surfaces per person, while 63 per cent of the elderly had root decay with a mean of 3.17 decayed and filled surfaces per person. In the longitudinal study referred to above, 47 per cent of the sample acquired new root caries lesions over the eighteen-month observation period.

Root caries is a significant problem in that it is difficult to treat clinically and restorations often fail. It is a significant cause of tooth loss in institutionalized older people who have high rates due to low levels of oral hygiene and the xerostomic effects of medications (Kitamura and Kiyak 1986).

Periodontal disease

Traditionally, periodontal disease was believed to be a progressive disorder, beginning as a marginal gingivitis and developing into periodontitis characterized by a cumulative and irreversible loss of periodontal attachment. This view of the disease was supported by the strong correlation between age and periodontal destruction. Current concepts suggest that gingivitis and periodontitis are distinct disorders and that periodontitis is not necessarily a progressive disorder: it may arrest at any stage, pass through active and quiescent phases, and involve stages in which there is healing. This view of periodontal disease has made more complex the interpretation of epidemiological data and projections made on the basis of that data.

Numerous studies have revealed that the elderly have the highest rates of gingival bleeding, calculus deposits and periodontal pocketing (Beck 1984). The national surveys recently completed in the US found that 68 per cent of the elderly sample had loss of periodontal attachment of 4 mm or more compared to 24 per cent of the sample of working age. There is also evidence to suggest that, in the presence of bacterial plaque, old people show a more rapid and severe inflammatory response than younger individuals. These data have been interpreted by some to mean that periodontal diseases will be an ever-increasing burden on society and the dental profession. However, there is evidence from the US that the prevalence and severity of periodontal disease in the population *as a whole* is declining at a fairly rapid rate, largely in response to improvements in oral hygiene. Certainly, the proportion of the population without any inflammatory disease rose markedly during the 1960s and 1970s. Given these observations, Page (1984) concludes that the high rate of periodontitis in the elderly represents a cohort rather than an aging effect so that the future elderly will have less rather than more periodontal disease.

Page's predictions are not as sound as they might appear. The reduction in periodontal disease in the US is almost wholly accounted for by a fall in the frequency of gingivitis. If this is not, as previously supposed, a precursor of periodontal disease then projections based on trends in gingivitis are diffficult to support. Clearly, the future problem posed by this group of disorders will remain uncertain until their natural history in different age groups has been clarified.

The elderly and the use of dental services

Although the elderly have high levels of need for dental care they tend, as a whole, to use dental services less frequently. They are less likely to have seen a dentist in the previous year and less likely to attend regularly for check-ups than younger age groups. Some of these differences are explained by the fact that many of the elderly are edentulous and perceive less need for dental care. If the utilization rates of the dentate elderly are compared with those for the rest of the adult population the differences are reduced considerably. In fact, one of the best predictors of a dental visit in the last year by the elderly is the retention of one or more natural teeth (Locker *et al.* 1987). Given the increasing likelihood of the elderly remaining dentate, demand for dental care should rise. This increase in utilization is already apparent in the US. The percentage of people aged 65 years and over visiting a dentist in the previous year rose from 21 per cent in 1963 to 43 per cent in 1981.

Other changes in the characteristics of the elderly population are likely to reinforce this trend of increasing demand. The 'new' elderly identified by Ettinger and Beck (1982) were better educated, and had higher incomes and more positive attitudes towards the natural dentition and dental care than the 'old' elderly. In fact, those aged 60 to 64 years were much more like the 18- to 59-year-olds in terms of these characteristics than those aged 65 years and over. Ettinger and Beck (1982) predict the evolution of a qualitatively different elderly consumer: more positively oriented to dental health, more politically aware and more demanding of health and social services. Whether the dental health care system is able to respond adequately to the collective and individual needs of these consumers will depend upon the development of policy initiatives directed at this previously neglected section of the population and upon the training and skills of the future generation of dental practitioners.

Problematic aspects of the dental care of the elderly

While the dental care needs and demands of the elderly are changing, other characteristics of the elderly population will remain stable. These are important since they complicate the delivery of optimal dental care to this group. The medical and functional status of elderly people is, perhaps, the most important factor which needs to be taken into account.

The elderly population is one in which there are large numbers of people who are medically compromised. Rates of chronic disabling disorders are high and conditions with implications for dental practice are particularly prevalent (Beck and Hunt 1985). Among the US population aged 65 years and over between 7 and 44 per cent are affected by diseases such as diabetes, hypertension, heart disease or arthritis. Sensory impairments also increase with age so that 12 per cent have a problem with vision and 28 per cent a problem with hearing (see Table 4.2).

Table 4.2 Prevalence of physical impairments, US: percentage by age group

Impairment	Age			
	<17	17–44	45–64	65+
Visual	1	3	6	12
Hearing	1	5	20	28
Speech	2	6	7	8
Paralysis of extremity	2	3	7	19

Source: Beck and Hunt 1985. Adapted

These disorders have one or both of the following consequences. First, they are frequently disabling and impede an individual's ability to perform the basic activities of daily living. For example, difficulties in walking are experienced by 19 per cent of those over the age of 65 and 10 per cent have difficulty in getting outside the house (NCHS 1987). Between 10 and 25 per cent of this population also have difficulty extending the arms above the shoulders, holding small objects or sitting comfortably for more than one hour. Table 4.3 gives the age-specific prevalence of disability for an inner city population in the UK.

Table 4.3 Prevalence of disability in an inner city community, UK: Percentage by age and sex

Age	Sex	Per cent
16–29	M	2.0
	F	2.3
30–49	M	4.6
	F	7.6
50–64	M	15.5
	F	16.3
65–74	M	25.2
	F	30.5
75 +	M	42.9
	F	58.6

Source: Patrick *et al.* 1981

Second, people with chronic disabling disorders are most likely taking one or more prescription medications. For example, in the US population, 75 per cent are taking at least one such drug and among those taking at least one the mean number per person is as high as 14 (NCHSR 1982). Beck and Hunt (1985) classified prescription medications into three groups, depending upon their dental effects. Class I drugs had a direct effect on the oral cavity, producing xerostomia or tissue hyperplasia; Class II drugs had an indirect effect, causing local or systemic complications for dental procedures, and Class III drugs had no known effects with respect to dental care. Using data from a national survey of medical care, they found that 81 per cent of people aged 65 and over were taking one or more drugs which fell into Class I or II.

When considering the provision of dental care, the elderly can be divided into three distinct groups: (1) those who are mobile and able to visit a dentist on their own initiative; (2) the homebound; and (3) the institutionalized. In general, the prevalence of chronic illness and disability will increase across these groups with the institutionalized being particularly disadvantaged. The main problem with regard to this group and the homebound is access to dental care. Mobility problems, problems with transportation, and the physical layout of the dental surgery are major barriers to dental treatment. If these groups of elderly are to receive treatment in line with their oral health care needs, then domiciliary visiting and the provision of care within institutions are essential (Smith *et al.* 1983). Given the visual and fine motor impairments characteristic of these elderly populations, one of their most basic needs is for assistance in maintaining optimal levels of oral hygiene. For this reason, hygienists are key members of the team providing care to the elderly.

Without doubt, diagnosis and treatment planning for the elderly patient present the dental practitioner with a challenge: both are more complex than is the case with younger patients. With the medically compromised elderly what seem to be simple oral complaints may be manifestations of more generalized systemic problems. Ettinger and Beck (1983) cite the example of an elderly denture wearer who presents with a sore mouth. They describe twelve possible diagnoses. The problem may be a localized one involving trauma or one that is linked to medications or underlying systemic conditions. If the complaint is a product of medication or other chronic disorders then diagnosis and treatment must proceed in consultation with the patient's physician and others involved in the provision of medical care.

Once a diagnosis has been made treatment planning is complicated by the many social, economic, and psychological factors which must be taken into account. The patient's life expectancy, future medical status and personal resources will all affect the type and timing of treatment provided. The main aim of treatment should be to remedy any overt oral or dental pathology and treat those conditions which are handicapping the patient in daily life (Smith *et al.* 1983). Ettinger and Beck (1983) describe this as 'rational' dental care. This is particularly the case with the frail elderly, whose needs for dental care are not determined solely by the presence of oral disease but based upon their ability to tolerate and benefit from dental treatment. While complex periodontal and restorative therapy may be appropriate for the active non-compromised individual, it may not be appropriate for those with chronic debilitating disorders. Because two people of the same age may be radically different in this regard, all decisions must be made on an individual basis. The attitudes and expectations of the patient's family or those providing care to the homebound or institutionalized may also need to be taken into account, for their cooperation is essential in maintaining and improving the oral health of the dependent elderly person. Their ability and willingness to assist with oral hygiene procedures may provide the key to treatment planning. While every effort should be made to preserve the natural dentition, extractions may be the treatment of choice for some patients. This is more likely to be the case with the patient who has gross dental lesions, a history of high susceptibility to dental disease, an oral cavity affected by medications, and an inability to achieve adequate levels of oral hygiene.

Because a proportion of the elderly population will present the dental practitioner with complex problems in diagnosis and treatment planning, continuity of care is essential. This means that any system providing for the needs of these patients must be structured in ways to facilitate such continuity.

Communication and the elderly patient

Communication is another factor which may complicate the provision of dental care for the elderly. Normal changes associated with aging and the presence of sensory impairments demand patience and sensitivity in managing the elderly patient (Geboy and Muzzio 1985). Many dentists find the elderly patient the least satisfying of all to treat and this may be related to difficulties in communication (Strayer *et al.* 1986). This in turn may be the product of negative attitudes towards the elderly and the belief that the elderly are less competent than younger adults and must be given overly simplistic explanations of their problems. This is often referred to as 'infantilization' and is likely to produce a negative response on the part of the elderly person, who quite rightly feels that his or her dignity has been compromised (Tamir 1979).

The dentist must also exercise special care and sensitivity in managing patients who are disabled. One major problem which occurs in relationships between people with and without disabilities is that of asking for and giving help. The physical assistance given to people with disabilities by their non-disabled counterparts can be unwelcome at best and demeaning at worst. The dentist and his or her staff should not assume that the person requires help but should ask what assistance is needed and how it might best be given. In this regard the patient rather than the dentist is the expert. The physical layout of the office is also a form of communication and, if constructed in ways which make access difficult for the elderly or disabled person, may be taken to indicate a lack of understanding of, or concern for, their needs.

Economic factors and the elderly person

A final factor that needs to be taken into account in the dental care of the elderly is their relatively low economic status. Households which are headed by a person over the age of 65 years have mean annual incomes which are less than half of households whose head is under the age of retirement. Moreover, the elderly in North America are the least likely to be covered by dental insurance schemes. There is no reason to believe that the purchasing power of the low-income elderly will improve as we move towards the next century. This may have fewer implications for publicly funded dental health care systems such as that in the UK than for the essentially private systems found in the US, Canada and Australia. Within the British system the elderly are likely to continue to receive free care even in the face of privatization of the General Dental Service by the progressive introduction of user charges. Within private systems pressure will grow for government intervention to make sure the elderly have access to the treatment they need. In order that publicly funded programmes are able to provide effective care at a price society is willing to pay, the dental profession may not have to accept innovative delivery systems and reimbursement mechanisms, such as capitation or payment by salary, which have traditionally received little in the way of support (see Chapter 14).

5

Measuring oral health: socio-dental indicators

The rational planning and evaluation of services to meet the health care needs of a population require data on the health status of that population and changes in health status over time. Such rational planning and evaluation have not played a prominent role in the development of health services in most industrialized nations. Rather, health care systems have evolved in piecemeal fashion and are often the product of historical accident, chance occurrence, or the response of communities to short-term need or transient political pressures. However, as the role of governments in the provision of health care has grown, the need for planning and evaluation has increased. As a consequence, interest in the measurement of health and the demand for data on the health status of populations have accelerated.

While government involvement in health care provision has stimulated interest in the measurement of health, a number of contemporary trends have reinforced and consolidated that interest. These include changes in the patterns of disease and illness in modern societies, changes in patterns of medical and dental practice, and the rising costs of health care provision. These historical trends have rendered the task of measuring the health status of populations both more necessary and more complex.

One of the major current concerns about health care is its rising costs. In most western nations the proportion of GNP spent on health has continued to grow. One of the reasons for rising costs has been the growth in the size and complexity of health care systems. Health care is labour-intensive: the National Health Service in the UK, for example, is Europe's largest employer. Other reasons include the rising demand for health care, particularly from aging populations (see Chapter 4), and the continuing growth in the use of expensive medical technology. As medical knowledge expands, so do the possibilities for, and costs of, treatment. However, the ability of the industrialized nations to spend more on health has been questioned. Efforts are now being made to cut costs and secure improvements in value for money. These efforts require a greater accountability on the part of those who spend health care resources, particularly with regard to the efficiency of services and treatments. Identifying opportunities for greater efficiency and monitoring the impact of cuts in expenditure means that data on health and the relationship between health and health services is needed.

Economic considerations have made the measurement of health more essential; changes in patterns of disease, illness, and attitudes to health have made such measurement more complex. The measurement of health status dates back to the mid-nineteenth century, when governments began to collect systematic data on death and the causes of death. These mortality statistics continue to be a major source of data about health. Mortality statistics, however, are only useful measures of health in populations where death rates are high. They are useful in developing countries where infant and maternal mortality rates are substantial and where short-term infectious and parasitic diseases remain major causes of death. In the industrialized nations, where death rates are low, mortality statistics and associated measures such as life expectancy are no longer adequate as indicators of health. They do not take account of illness that does not result in death and ignore the often profound disability and distress that accompany such illness. Largely as a result of social and environmental change, the infectious diseases that used to be major causes of death have been replaced by the modern epidemics of cancer, heart disease and chronic, disabling disorders (see Chapter 1). These diseases are long term, largely incurable, impose a profound social and psychological burden on the individual and family, and result in a radically reduced quality of life. Accordingly, contemporary definitions of health have broadened: health is now recognized to be multidimensional and to involve not only the presence or absence of disease but also its social and psychological consequences. Along with contemporary concerns with the quality of life, this broader definition has made the measurement of health more difficult. We must now take account of physical, social, and psychological realities.

One of the first definitions to acknowledge the multidimensional nature of health was formulated by the World Health Organization in 1948. Health was defined as 'a complete state of physical, mental and social well-being and not merely the absence of illness'. While this definition has been criticized because it represents an unattainable ideal and is not easily operationalized into a measure, it does indicate that health involves sociomedical as well as biophysical concerns. More recently, other related concepts have been refined and a basic distinction drawn between disease and illness (Field 1976, Culyer 1983). The former refers to medically defined abnormalities in anatomical structures or physiological or biochemical processes, while the latter refers to the individual's experience or subjective perception of changes in physical and mental well-being (Hunt *et al.* 1986). Accordingly, measuring health means that clinical indices which assess the presence or severity of pathological conditions need to be supplemented by measures of the subjective aspects of health. These measures, based on social and psychological functioning and self-perceived feeling states, document the immediate personal and broader social consequences of disease.

Measures of oral health status

The medical literature on the measurement of health status is extensive, and a wide variety of clinical and sociomedical measures have been developed for use in research and policy formulation (Scrivens *et al.* 1985, Hunt *et al.* 1986). This literature has yet to be matched by a comparable one in dentistry. While a great deal of effort has been devoted to the construction of valid and reliable indices of oral disease, behavioural or subjective measures of oral health have rarely been used: dentistry has remained narrowly clinical in its conception and understanding of oral health.

There are a number of reasons why dentistry has remained relatively immune to contemporary concepts of health. These include differences in the nature of physical and oral disorders and in approaches to patient management, the extent to which the behavioural sciences have contributed to dental health care research, and the perceptions of researchers themselves. The last reason is one of the most important, for even where consideration has been given to the social and psychological consequences of dental and oral conditions, it has often been assumed that they are either non-existent or negligible. For example, Davis (1976), in a major theoretical statement, has argued that the impact of dental and oral disease on daily life is minimal. He claims that these diseases are not life threatening and do not give rise to the changes in behaviour observed in relation to more serious disorders. Davis's view has recently been challenged by research which has demonstrated that dental and oral diseases are not inconsequential; they impose a significant burden both on the individual and the community (see Chapter 6).

The measures currently employed to document the dental and oral health status of populations, such as the DMF Index and Russell's Periodontal Index, are measures of existing or past dental disease. They assess and quantify the presence and extent of damage to the teeth and their supporting structures as a result of oral pathological processes. In the case of measures such as the CPITN (Community Periodontal Index of Treatment Needs), clinical assessments are converted into indices of treatment needs. As measures of oral health, these indices are not above criticism. The DMFT Index, which is intended to measure caries experience, is subject to a number of well-known limitations (Burt 1983). It is often difficult, for example, to be sure that filled and missing teeth, particularly in adults, have not been filled or lost for reasons other than decay. Consequently, its validity as an indicator of caries experience is subject to some doubt.

From the point of view of contemporary definitions of health, however, such measures are subject to more serious limitations; they tell us nothing about the functioning of either the oral cavity or the person as a whole and nothing about subjectively perceived symptoms such as pain and discomfort. Even more complex measures such as Helkimo's anamnestic and clinical indices of temporomandibular joint disorders (Helkimo 1974) are problematic in this regard. While the severity of joint and muscle pain and limitations in the mobility of the mandible are assessed in classifying patients with disorders of the masticatory system, their impact on everyday activities such as eating and talking is not. Clinical indices of the kind mentioned are, of course, essential to the task of measuring oral disease; the problem arises when these indices are treated as measures of health and treatment need (Sheiham *et al.* 1982).

Socio-dental indicators

The limitations of current measures of oral disorders have been recognized in recent discussions of oral disease and the quality of life. These have noted the lack of systematic data on the social and psychological impact of such disease on individuals and societies (Cohen and Jago 1976, Nikias *et al.* 1979, Nikias 1985, Reisine 1985). A recent review of research in this field shows that only acute dental episodes, malocclusion, and dento-facial anomalies have received any attention with regard to their social and psychological outcomes and even this research is relatively sparse (Reisine 1984). Yet as Nikias (1985) states, measurement of the consequences of these diseases is essential to a full scientific understanding of the scope of oral health problems, rational decision-making with regard to the allocation of health care resources, and the evaluation of dental health services.

These discussions of clinical indices and oral health recommend the construction and use of socio-dental indicators. These are measures of the extent to which dental and oral disorders disrupt normal social-role functioning and bring about major changes in behaviour such as an inability to work or attend school, or undertake parental or household duties. The major research effort in this field has been concerned with days of work lost as a result of dental and oral disorders. Clearly, work loss can have an impact on the individual in the form of loss of wages and an impact on society as a whole in terms of lost productivity and its effect on the national economy. Reisine and Miller (1986) have shown that at the level of the individual work loss due to these disorders is small: a mean of 1.26 hours per year. However, if this figure is multiplied by the total number of people employed, work loss at a national level becomes substantial. As data presented in Chapter 6 show, it has been estimated that 7.1 million days of work are lost each year in the US as a result of dental disease.

Clearly, work loss days are a useful indicator of the impact of dental disorders on society as a whole, but would not be a sensitive indicator at the level of the individual. A comprehensive understanding of the consequences of oral disease requires a broad range of measures and indicators able to assess the effect of oral disease on individuals and communities. Measures are required which are sensitive enough to detect the often subtle, although significant, changes in well-being caused by dental and oral disease. Measures which are confined to major changes in role behaviour, such as

Table 5.1 Health status concepts and measures

Concept/Category	Definition
BIOPHYSICAL	
1 Death	Mortality rates, life expectancy, potential years of life lost
2 Disease	
(i) Self-report	Patient listings of diagnoses or medical conditions
(ii) Clinical diagnoses	Diagnoses found on clinical examination
3 Impairment	Extent of anatomical loss or structural abnormality
4 Functional limitation	Extent of loss of function of body parts or systems
SOCIOMEDICAL	
1 Discomfort	Self-reported physical and psychological distress, including pain and other feeling states not directly observable
2 Disability	
(i) Physical well-being	
Activity restriction	Acute or chronic limitation in physical activities of daily living
Limitations in social roles	Acute or chronic problems in work, school, household management and recreation
(ii) Psychological well-being	
Affective states	Emotional states, anxiety, depression
Cognitive states	Problems in concentration, reasoning
(iii) Social well-being	
Integration	Participation in community life
Social contacts	Interaction with family, friends
Intimacy	Perceived feelings of closeness/support
3 Disadvantage	
(i) Inequality of opportunity	Lack of access to social opportunities, including careers, education
(ii) Deprivation	Inequality of outcomes in terms of income, self-image, self-esteem
(iii) Dissatisfaction	With health and/or overall quality of life

work loss, are inadequate because they do not take account of the many experiential and psychological outcomes of oral disease.

A conceptual framework

The main problem involved in developing a comprehensive set of measures of oral health is deciding precisely what should be measured. What kind of events can be identified as indicating health and ill-health? Guidance can be found in a comprehensive set of concepts defined by Wood (1980) and Patrick (1982). Wood's framework consists of the concepts of impairment, functional limitation, disability and handicap. These identify distinct areas of human experience relative to diseases and its personal and social consequences. Accordingly, it links concepts drawn from medicine and the behavioural sciences to capture a broad spectrum of events, each of which provides the basis for specific types of health status measure. Although it was originally applied to chronic disabling diseases, the scheme is applicable to all physical, psychological and oral disorders. Patrick (1982) has described an overlapping and somewhat broader range of concepts which provides the basis for the measurement of health status. These are: death, disease, disability, discomfort, and dissatisfaction. Like the concepts defined by Wood (1980), these involve both biological concerns and concerns with the quality of life. In everyday practice dentists and physicians apply such concepts, either implicitly or explicitly, during their evaluations of patients and treatment needs. The concepts are summarized in Table 5.1 and their application to dentistry and dental disorders is discussed below.

Categories and concepts of health

Death

Death, despite its limitations, is an essential concept in assessing the health of populations. Death rates, life expectancy and potential years of life lost, for example, are used as indicators of health and societal well-being. Death is an important outcome of many diseases and can be useful as a measure of the relative success of alternative treatment modalities or in comparisons of the relative disadvantage of nations or groups. At the level of the individual, death is a readily observable and unequivocal outcome. Moreover, in most developed societies, data on mortality are routinely collected and readily available. In many respects, the debate over the adequacy of mortality rates as measures of health is irrelevant to dentistry. Although oral cancers are a significant cause of death, accounting for 9000 deaths in the US in 1980 (Sheiham and Croog 1981), death rates are not a useful indicator or measure of the impact of the more common dental and oral disorders.

Disease

Disease, impairment and functional limitation are closely allied concepts which refer to pathological processes affecting the psychological or physical make-up of human individuals. Here, disease is taken to be a label applied to these pathological processes and, as such, is measured in terms of its frequency in populations. The two most common ways of estimating prevalence and incidence rates are based on clinical diagnoses or self-reported diagnoses. The former may be collected routinely or acquired by means of population surveys, while the latter are always survey-based and used where clinical assessment of large numbers of individuals is not possible. Estimates of the prevalence of major disabling conditions, for example, are almost always based on self-report data, despite some doubt as to their validity. Routinely collected morbidity data are limited to a relatively narrow range of diseases. Sources of information include cancer registrations, infectious disease reports and hospital discharge data. Such data vary in quality, they are usually biased, and limited to treated populations. Some data on dental disorders are routinely collected in the UK and some provinces of Canada where publicly funded dental health services or publicly administered insurance schemes are in place. Unfortunately, they tell us more about treatments provided than disease. Data on the prevalence and incidence of oral disorders are almost always derived from clinical examinations undertaken as part of population surveys which use the familiar dental health indices to estimate the proportion of the population with common oral disorders.

Impairment

Impairment is defined as any anatomical loss, structural

abnormality or disturbance in physical or psychological processes, either present at birth or arising out of disease or injury. Measures of impairment give an indication of the nature and extent of anatomical loss or structural abnormality associated with disease, injury or birth defects. Such measures are common within dentistry. Edentulism, number of remaining functional units and the M component of the DMFT index are measures of tissue loss, while the many schemes for classifying malocclusion describe the type and sometimes the extent of structural abnormalities of the teeth and jaws. The many systems for assessing periodontal disease also provide quantitative estimates of the presence and extent of damage to the periodontium.

Functional limitation

Functional limitation completes the set of concepts necessary for the measurement of disease and its biophysical consequences. Functional limitations are defined as restrictions in the functions customarily expected of the body or its component organs or systems. Measures of functional limitation are less common in dentistry but still widely used. For example, assessments of limitations of jaw mobility, including restricted opening and restricted lateral and protrusive movements, are used in classifying the severity of temporomandibular dysfunction. Similarly, indices of chewing efficiency measure the functional limitation arising out of oral disease.

Discomfort

The remaining concepts listed in Table 5.1 give rise to scales and indices which are usually grouped under the general heading 'sociomedical measures'. These broaden considerably the assessment of health and address areas given increasing importance in medical care. They do not replace the traditional biomedical measures; rather, they extend such measures to enhance our understanding of human beings and their responses to disease (Hunt and McEwen 1980). They include assessments of restrictions in activity and subjective appraisals of well-being. At the very end of the continuum these health status measures begin to merge with measures of the quality of life.

Self-reported pain and discomfort, physical and psychological symptoms and other not directly observable feeling states are sometimes used as proxy measures of disease and sometimes as measures in their own right. Some would regard pain as an indicator of an underlying pathological process (Patrick 1982) while others would regard pain as a psychological consequence of disease (Nikias 1985). Here discomfort is treated as a sociomedical measure because it is subjectively perceived and may be experienced even in the absence of an underlying clinical condition. This conforms to the current view that disease and illness are distinct realities and an individual can be or feel ill without being diseased (Field 1976). While pain is probably the most common symptom of oral and dental disorders, systematic data on the prevalence of acute and chronic oro-facial pain are currently lacking.

Disability

Disability is a behavioural concept and defined as any limitation in or lack of ability to perform the activities of daily living. While early measures of disability focused upon a narrow range of such activities, most frequently mobility, body movement and self-care, current approaches encompass the distinct dimensions of physical, psychological and social well-being. The most comprehensive and sensitive measure in current use is the Sickness Impact Profile (SIP) developed in the US (Bergner and Bobbitt 1981). This uses 136 items to measure the effect of disease on 12 major aspects of daily living. An impression of the scope of this instrument can be gained from Table 5.2, which lists its 12 constituent categories.

Physical well-being is made up of two components: *activity restrictions* consist of acute or chronic limitations in such areas of life as ambulation, mobility, self-care, eating, and sleep and rest; while *limitations in usual social roles* involve problems in work, household management and recreation. Contemporary measures of disability differ according to whether they cover these components and the extent to which they do so, although the more comprehensive indices, such as the Sickness Impact Profile, include a number of sub-scales relative to each.

Reduced ability to carry out the activities of daily living is a concept equally applicable to individuals and populations. Because measures such as the SIP are very detailed and time-consuming to apply, they are more readily used on individuals or small samples.

Table 5.2 Sickness impact profile categories

Dimension	Items describing behaviour related to:
PHYSICAL	Ambulation
	Mobility
	Body care and movement
	Sleep and rest
	Eating
PSYCHOSOCIAL	Social interaction
	Alertness behaviour
	Emotional behaviour
	Communication
SOCIAL ROLES	Work
	Home management
	Recreation and pastimes

In assessing the physical well-being of populations, cruder measures are necessary, especially when the data are collected on an on-going basis as in the British General Household Survey and the US National Health Survey Days of restricted activity, work-disability days and bed-disability days are used to document the impact of illness. Where such behaviours can be attributed to dental or oral conditions, then the measures constitute what have been referred to as sociodental indicators.

Since psychological and social well-being are equally likely to be affected by disease, they are now given due attention in assessments of disability. Of six major measures reviewed by Verkleij and Spruit (1984), only one did not address social and emotional health. Disease may affect psychological processes in two ways. First, it may give rise to changes in emotional and affective states, all of which involve distress. Anxiety, depression, uncertainty, emotional fatigue, loss of volition and feelings of hopelessness are common complaints among those with chronic conditions. Cognitive functioning may also be affected and result in confusion, forgetfulness, an inability to make decisions, and problems in thought and concentration. In the context of dentistry, acute and chronic pain are most likely to have these effects.

Measures of social well-being need to include social integration, social contacts, and social and emotional intimacy. The first is concerned with the extent of an individual's participation in community life and is assessed on the basis of membership of formal and informal organizations. The second is concerned with the frequency of interaction with friends and relatives and the third with the quality of those interactions, assessed in terms of the presence of one or more individuals who provide psychosocial and instrumental support. Clearly, many diseases, including acute and chronic dental disorders, can have a temporary or permanent impact on all three.

Handicap

While disability refers to the immediate personal consequences of disease, handicap is concerned with its broader social effects. Handicap is defined as the disadvantage experienced by impaired and disabled people because they do not or cannot conform to the expectations of society or the social groups to which they belong. Any loss or abnormality of structure or function, or the behavioural limitations involved, can have an effect on both the quality of everyday life and long-term life chances.

Detailed descriptions of the many forms of disadvantage experienced by chronically sick or disabled people are quite common. Measures of disadvantage, however, are rarely to be found in the literature. One problem is that disadvantage is also multidimensional and can involve loss of opportunity, actual material and social deprivation, and dissatisfaction. Disease and disability can have a negative effect on marriage and family formation, employment prospects, income, self-image and self-esteem, and loneliness and social isolation. Some of these effects have been reported with respect to dental and oral disease. These diseases, either directly or because of their relationship to physical attractiveness, have been shown to affect the social acceptability and school performance of children (Shaw *et al.* 1980a). Similarly, people with facial clefts are more likely to remain single, marry later in life or have childless marriages (Peter and Chinsky 1974). Clearly, the nature and extent of disadvantage experienced will vary according to the specific condition and its characteristics. Capturing these effects by means of a single measure will be difficult. Currently, measures of the quality of life are the best indicators of disadvantage and deprivation (Andrews and Withey 1974).

A conceptual model

As shown in Figure 5.1, these concepts are linked in a linear fashion to produce an overall scheme which moves from a biological to a behavioural, and then social, level of analysis. This model is an adaptation of that recently adopted by the WHO as part of the *International Classification of Impairments, Disabilities and Handicaps* (1980). The diagram also illustrates the various relationships between the component parts of the overall model. For example, handicap may be the outcome of a linear progression along the full sequences of events depicted. Rheumatoid arthritis provides a good illustration of this. The disease affects the supporting tissue of joints, which then become painful, weakened, and limited in their range of movement. This imposes severe restrictions on the individual's ability to perform the basic activities of daily living, leading in many cases to unemployment, poverty, social isolation and a psychologically debilitating dependence on others. This disorder demonstrates that disability may be a product of discomfort as well as functional limitations. Even before rheumatoid arthritis has damaged the joints themselves, the chronic pain associated with the condition can be severely disabling (Locker 1983).

Figure 5.1 The conceptual model

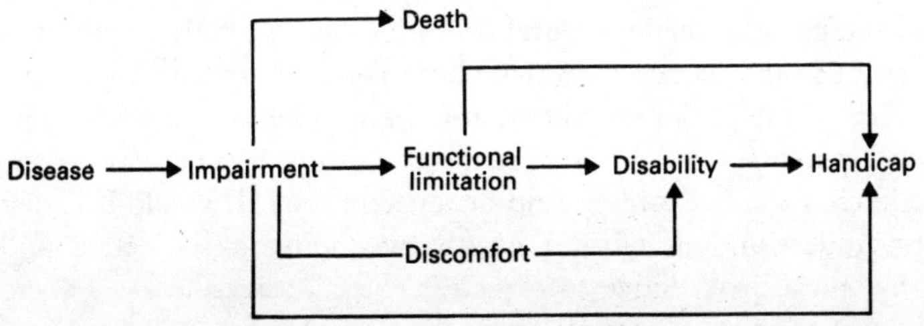

Source: WHO 1980. Adapted

Handicap may also be the product of conditions which involve functional limitations but do not cause disability. Wood (1980) quotes the case of an individual with coeliac disease who is able to lead a normal life in terms of daily activities but who may be disadvantaged by the need to follow a special and expensive diet.

Finally, handicap may result from conditions which are neither functionally limiting nor disabling, as in the case of a facial disfigurement which causes embarrassment and other problems in relationships with others.

That this dynamic model is applicable to dental and oral conditions is readily illustrated by reference to a recent paper by Smith and Sheiham (1979) concerning the oral health problems of the elderly. Because many of the elderly they interviewed were continuing to manage with poor and ill-fitting dentures, edentulism (impairment), largely the result of caries and periodontitis (disease), resulted in difficulties in chewing (functional limitation) which in turn restricted their ability to eat (disability). Many were unable to eat foods of their choice, and many found that it took much longer for them to complete a meal. This detracted from the pleasure of eating, caused embarrassment, and deterred them from eating with others (handicap). Many also reported social discomfort because of the poor appearance of their dentition and difficulties with talking and singing. In this way, dental and oral conditions have a negative impact on the quality of life and lead to various forms of social and psychological deprivation.

Properties of socio-dental measures

Measures and indicators of the discomfort, disability and disadvantage associated with oral conditions are urgently required to document the extent to which these conditions impinge on the quality of life of the individual and the well-being of society. The development of a valid and reliable measure comparable to the Sickness Impact Profile would be a useful start. It would broaden our understanding of oral health by adding a subjective and behavioural perspective to objective clinical assessments. Taking account of these events conforms with contemporary concepts of health, expands the definition of need used in dentistry (Sheiham *et al.* 1982), provides a more comprehensive basis for the monitoring of individual and societal welfare, and offers additional measures to be used in the evaluation of dental health care.

However, the task does not end there, for the next challenge is to develop further the model presented in Figure 5.1 in order to discover the complex relationships between its component parts. These relationships are not direct: impairment does not necessarily lead to disability any more than disability necessarily results in disadvantage. While these outcomes are dependent upon the nature and severity of the disorder they are also modified by social and psychological variables. Research on rehabilitation has shown that the level of disability that results from a chronic disorder is influenced by a number of these variables, including self-perception, family background and social support. Similarly, social and financial resources and the psychological capacity to cope with illness and disability influence the extent of social disadvantage experienced (Locker 1983). Dental disease will have less impact on the income of the upper as opposed to the lower socio-economic groups, particularly where dental services are not free or dental insurance schemes not universally available, and facial clefts will have less of an impact on those with the psychological capacity to cope with awkwardness in social encounters. Exploring the links between clinical conditions and their personal and social outcomes not only promotes a more complex appreciation of oral health, it also provides the opportunity to identify interventions to minimize the consequences of this important group of diseases. In this way, such knowledge contributes directly to patient well-being.

6
The social and psychological consequences of oral disease

Oral health has often been accorded low priority by governments and health care policy makers. While most developed countries provide dental services for the more vulnerable members of the community, for example, children, the elderly, the handicapped and the poor, few have comprehensive, publicly funded oral health care systems. In countries such as Canada, where medical care is provided by compulsory, universal health insurance schemes, dental care for most adults must be purchased out of their own pockets or financed by means of occupationally linked or voluntary dental insurance plans. Even in countries such as the UK, where dentistry is part of the National Health Service, dental care is under-financed and increasingly subject to user fees. In short, in most industrialized nations, adult dental health is only rarely viewed as a significant public health issue (Miller 1987).

Perhaps because dental and oral disorders are only infrequently life-threatening, it is easy to assume that dental health and dentistry contribute little to overall individual and societal welfare. The aim of this chapter is to demonstrate that this is not the case: dental and oral disorders have significant social, psychological and economic consequences and a significant impact on the quality of life. If dental disorders are regarded as trivial and undeserving of public concern, it is because we have neglected to measure, and make policy makers aware of, these consequences. As noted in the previous chapter, our approach to dental disease has been narrowly clinical and relatively little attention has been paid to the extent to which these diseases disable and handicap. Systematic and quantitative information on the impact of oral disease is essential to decisions about the allocation of scarce health care resources. It also provides the practitioner with a comprehensive understanding of the oral disease and its consequences for the individual patient. Using the conceptual framework outlined in the previous chapter, there follows a summary of research which has addressed these issues, both at the level of the individual and of the community as a whole.

Discomfort

Pain and discomfort are common consequences of oral disorders and likely to have an immediate and significant impact on the quality of life. Until recently, however, very little was known about the prevalence of such pain and discomfort in the population. An early study in the UK obtained data from 236 women and their husbands, and found that 7.5 per cent reported having toothache in the previous four weeks. Using data on the duration of the pain, it was estimated that dental pain occurred on three days per person per year, amounting to 200 million days of pain for the UK as a whole (Miller *et al.* 1975). A more recent study of employed adults in England found 26 per cent had dental pain and 50 per cent oral discomfort during the previous year (Cushing *et al.* 1986). Similarly, a survey of a representative sample of adults in the US found that 27 per cent had experienced dental pain in the year prior to interview. Studies of chronic pain have also been reported in the literature. Basker *et al.* (1978) found 2.6 per cent of the patients attending five general practices in the UK reported the prolonged burning pain characteristic of Burning Mouth Syndrome, and studies from Scandinavia and Hungary suggest that 7 to 12 per cent of the population have pain associated with temporomandibular joint dysfunction.

Two more detailed studies of oral pain and discomfort have been undertaken in Canada. A mail survey of a random sample of 594 adults living in the City of Toronto asked questions about a variety of types of oral pain and discomfort (Locker and Grushka 1987a). Overall, 40 per cent experienced one or more pain symptoms in the previous four weeks. Those most commonly reported were pain in the teeth with hot or cold fluids or sweet things (29 per cent) and toothache (14 per cent) (see Table 6.1). Questions about the severity of the pain revealed that four per cent of the *entire sample* had experienced severe pain in the four weeks prior to the completion of the questionnaire while 15 per cent had

Table 6.1 Prevalence of oral and facial pain: percentage reporting pain in the previous four weeks

Pain in the teeth with hot or cold fluids or sweet things	29%
Toothache	14%
Pain in the jaw joints	9%
Pain in the face just in front of the ear	9%
Pain in the jaw while chewing	8%
Pain in the jaw joint while opening the mouth wide	6%
Sharp shooting pains across the face or cheeks	5%
A prolonged burning sensation in the tongue or other parts of the mouth	4%

Source: Locker and Grushka 1987a

experienced pain of moderate severity. In addition, 27 per cent reported discomfort from dentures, oral ulcerations or recurrent herpetic lesions, or sore and bleeding gums during the same period. The same set of questions was used in an oral health survey of persons living in East York, Ontario and found pain prevalence rates identical to those obtained from the mail survey.

The second study involved a telephone survey of a random sample of 677 adults drawn from the same population. This was concerned with the pain and other symptoms associated with temporomandibular disorders. One or more of the nine symptoms were reported by 48.4 per cent of those interviewed. Pain was reported by 13 per cent and non-pain symptoms such as joint sounds, intermittent locking, limited mouth opening and stiffness or tenderness of masticatory muscles by 36 per cent. One quarter of those with pain judged it to be moderately severe or severe and 13 per cent of those with other symptoms were bothered by them to a significant degree (Locker and Slade 1988).

The mail survey of oral pain described above found that pain was more common in the younger than the older age groups. This is largely because the majority of pain episodes are associated with the teeth and the elderly are less likely to be dentate. Nevertheless, some studies have found high rates of pain in elderly populations and a high prevalence of other, equally distressing, symptoms. In a study of elderly people living at home, Smith and Sheiham (1979) found that 32 per cent complained of pain. The majority of these had intermittent pain, a quarter had pain while eating and five subjects were in constant pain. In four fifths of these cases, the pain was due to wearing a clinically unsatisfactory denture. Among the elderly studied by Berkey *et al.* (1985), 40 per cent complained of a dry mouth and 11 per cent of taste changes in the mouth.

The conceptual framework presented in the previous chapter suggests that pain in and of itself can be disabling. Evidence of the impact of oral pain on behaviour was obtained from the mail survey of adults in Toronto. The behaviour changes reported by those experiencing pain are listed in Table 6.2. The numbers reporting a behavioural impact have been expressed as a percentage of those having pain and as a percentage of the respondents as a whole. The latter gives an estimate of the burden imposed by oral pain on the community at large. As the table shows, almost 15 per cent of the population reported that oral pain had some effect on daily life in the four weeks in question. In the study of temporomandibular problems, half of those reporting pain, or 6 per cent of the sample as a whole, had difficulty eating, talking or swallowing.

Table 6.2 Behavioural consequences of oral and facial pain; pain subgroup and total sample

	Pain subgroup	Total sample
Took time off from work	4.2	1.7
Stayed in bed more than usual	4.1	1.5
Stayed home more than usual	5.2	2.0
Avoided family and friends	7.7	3.0
Sleep disturbance	14.2	5.5
Changed diet	30.6	11.9
One or more of the above	36.9	14.5

Source: Locker and Grushka 1987b

Disability

The disabling effects of dental and oral disorders are best described using the 12 life domains which comprise the Sickness Impact Profile (see Table 5.2). Most of the research in this area has been concerned with eating, work, and the emotional consequences of oral conditions, although some data are also available on sleep disturbance, social interaction and recreational activity. Although by no means systematic or comprehensive, these data, along with information on the prevalence of oral symptoms, clearly demonstrate the pervasive consequences of dental and oral conditions.

Work loss and overall social functioning

In population surveys the impact of disease on social functioning is measured in terms of days of restricted activity, bed disability days and days of work loss. The first consists of days on which an individual cuts down on his/her usual activities, the second of days on which a person spends all or most of the time in bed, and the third of days when an individual is absent from work (or school) for more than half a day. Reisine (1985) used data from the US National Health Survey to show that in 1981 4.9 million acute dental conditions were reported and caused 17.7 million days of restricted activity, 6.7 million days of bed disability and 7.1 million days of work loss. Compared to other equally common disorders such as gastrointestinal conditions, dental disorders had a relatively greater impact, with one and a half days of work lost for each condition reported. Ettinger (1987) used more recent data to compare the disabling effects of a range of common conditions and found that dental disease caused as many if not more problems than many of these other conditions (Table 6.3).

Table 6.3 Number of days of disability associated with a variety of acute conditions measured as a ratio of per 100 persons per year

Acute condition	Restricted activity	Bed days	Work loss
Dental conditions	7.4	2.4	3.1
Pneumonia	22.0	13.2	3.5
Acute eye conditions	1.6	0.9	0.3
Acute ear conditions	16.2	6.6	2.2
Acute urinary conditions	12.0	7.1	2.5
Skin conditions	6.8	2.3	1.6
Headache	4.8	2.4	1.2

Source: Ettinger 1987

Reisine also compared dental conditions with two more serious disorders, neoplasms and stroke. While the impact of these diseases on the individual and family is profound, the results were striking in that dental conditions caused twice as many work loss days as stroke and only half as many as neoplasms. Moreover, work loss due to dental conditions was concentrated in the younger age groups when productive capacity is at its highest. Clearly, oral conditions have a major effect on productivity and the economic well-being of society.

In order to overcome the limitations in the data produced by the National Health Survey, Reisine and Miller (1986) undertook a special study of work loss associated with dental disorders. Over a period of a year 26 per cent of the 2500 subjects interviewed were absent from work due to dental conditions or dental visits associated with those conditions. Most of these reported half a day or less of work loss, although 13 per cent reported one day or more. The average amount of work loss over the sample as a whole was small, only 1.26 hours per year per person. However, when multiplied by the size of the labour force for the US, work loss due to dental disorders becomes substantial. The study also suggested that regular preventive visits minimized the amount of time lost from work.

A study of college students also found that the symptoms associated with one particular oral condition affected daily functioning (Solberg *et al.* 1979). A quarter of a substantial sample of students reported symptoms of TMJ disorder and half of these found them problematic. Pain, headaches, and sleep loss were common and highly likely to interfere with studying and other educational activities. Another study found that dental problems had an adverse effect on the academic performance of a group of Indian schoolgirls aged 9 to 14 years (Koshi 1971).

Eating and nutrition

Eating is one of the most important functions of the oral cavity. It is a significant biological and social activity, and contributes enormously to individual well-being. Because the numbers of elderly in the population are increasing, the relationship between oral health, eating, and nutrition is an area of growing research interest to both gerontologists and dentists. Although eating problems are more likely to occur in the elderly, largely due to their increased prevalence of tooth loss and edentulism, it is by no means confined to this section of the population. Cushing *et al.* (1986) found that 20 per cent of their sample of persons aged 16–60 reported problems with eating. This varied from one in seven of the dentate to one in two of full denture wearers. Similarly, Locker and Grushka (1987b) found that 11 per cent of a population sample changed some aspect of their diet in response to dental or oral pain.

It has been estimated that the chewing efficiency of denture wearers is approximately 12 per cent of that of people with natural teeth. Consequently, denture wearers of all ages are more likely to report problems chewing foods. Most attention, however, has been focused on the elderly, since high rates of edentulism and associated medical problems make them a particularly vulnerable group. Among this section of the population around one third experience some difficulty chewing foods (Cushing *et al.* 1986). Among elderly denture wearers this may rise to almost 70 per cent (Locker *et al.* 1987). Problems with chewing often lead to an alteration in the foods that the elderly choose to eat. Solid or fibrous foods, or foods that slip easily under dentures are avoided and foods of softer consistency substituted. Twelve per cent of those studied by Cushing and Sheiham had changed the foods they ate or their methods of cooking them. In turn, such food substitution in the diet may have one or more outcomes. It may have nutritional outcomes in terms of the overall adequacy of the diet, or it may have negative social and psychological outcomes which impinge directly on the quality of life.

Dietary assessments among the elderly indicate that their dietary pattern differs from that of younger people. Older Americans consume more milk products, cereals, pasta, fruit, sugars and sweets than younger adults, and eat less meat, poultry, fish and vegetables (Peterkin *et al.* 1987). The diets of elderly denture wearers tend to differ from the diets of those who retain their natural teeth. They consume more calories in the form of carbohydrates and fats, and fewer proteins; they are more likely to have a lower than recommended intake of iron, thiamine, and riboflavin.

In spite of these differences, it is probably the case that the majority of the edentulous elderly have an adequate nutritional intake, although this is difficult to evaluate, given the lack of research on the nutrient requirements of old people. Similarly, the role of oral health status in food selection and nutrition is also complicated by sociodemographic factors such as poverty or low education. The social and psychological outcomes of poor chewing ability and limited food selection are, however, easier to assess and may be more significant to the individual concerned than the problems posed by a lower than recommended intake of various foods and nutrients.

Although the primary function of food is biological, eating is a complex set of activities with many social, psychological, and even religious ramifications. In almost all known societies, food is used to maintain and develop social relationships, so that an inability to participate fully in eating is experienced as a significant loss (Epstein 1987). In some cultures, food plays such an important social or religious role that it is vital to psychological health. Food is also a significant source of pleasure and may be relatively more so for the elderly to whom so many other sources of gratification are denied. For those with poor oral health, the choice may be one of continuing to eat foods that are enjoyed or valued, often in the face of pain or discomfort, or accepting a diet that produces little in the way of personal satisfaction. One source of satisfaction in eating is taste. There is some evidence to suggest that denture wearers do not have the ability of dentate persons to differentiate between foods of different levels of sweetness. This lack of taste discrimination may itself influence food choice.

One fifth of the edentulous elderly interviewed by Locker *et al.* (1987) said that they were prevented from eating foods they enjoyed because of problems with their teeth and mouth. Even the dentate were not spared: 11 per cent reported the same problem. Other difficulties arising out of poor chewing ability have been described by Smith and Sheiham (1979). One tenth of their sample felt uncomfortable eating in front of others and two fifths found that they took a long time to complete a meal. This caused embarrassment for many and meant that they preferred to eat alone. Ettinger (1987) has suggested that these coping mechanisms ultimately lead to social isolation and depression.

Although the links between masticatory ability, diet, eating, and the quality of dentures have not been studied to any great extent, the data indicate that many of these problems are avoided by the provision of satisfactory dentures. It should be noted that only 10 per cent of those studied by Smith and Sheiham had dentures that were clinically acceptable.

Because an inability to chew adequately leads to the swallowing of large food boluses, poor mastication has been linked to gastrointestinal discomfort and gastric disease. Much of the evidence for this is anecdotal and epidemiological studies have been too poor in terms of design to be able to clarify the issue. Hunt (1985), in a study of 3600 elderly people, found that those who had lost all their teeth were no more likely to report a history of gastric ulcer or digestive problems when compared to their dentate counterparts. However, edentulous persons with adequate prosthetic replacements may be able to chew more efficiently than dentate persons who retain only a few natural teeth. Since no data were obtained on masticatory function, the impact of chewing problems on gastric disease could not be properly explored in this study.

Social interaction

Another major function of the oral cavity is verbal and non-verbal communication. In spite of its importance, very little research has assessed the extent of difficulties in communication caused by oral health problems. However, the evidence that is available indicates that a minority of people do experience problems in this area. For example, in the study of persons aged 50 years and over by Locker *et al.* (1987), two per cent of subjects were dissatisfied with their ability to speak and eight per cent said they avoided smiling or laughing because of the appearance or health of their mouth. Almost a third were dissatisfied with the appearance of their teeth or dentures and 14 per cent reported that their appearance had caused them embarrassment. However, relatively few said that they had ever avoided meeting people socially because of this. Problems connected with the appearance of the teeth were more common among those who retained natural teeth. Obviously, these are more likely to be malaligned, irregularly spaced, stained, filled, or subject to gingival recession than prosthetic replacements. This helps to explain why more edentulous than dentate elderly say they are satisfied with their oral health status (Ranta *et al.* 1987).

Emotional and psychological functioning

Worry, fear, and anxiety are probably the most prevalent consequences of oral disorders. They may be provoked by oral symptoms and the person's concerns about their short- and long-term clinical and economic implications, or they may be provoked by the thought of having to undergo dental treatment. Fear and anxiety are major barriers to dental care and complicate the management of patients during treatment. The problems they create for the delivery of dental care are discussed in Chapters 9 and 10. Worry and concern about oral health per se were observed in 59 per cent of a sample of Canadian subjects aged 50 years and over (Locker *et al.* 1987) and in 62 per cent of a random sample of this population (Locker and Grushka 1987b). Among those experiencing pain, these psychological outcomes were reported by 70 per cent, most of whom said they had been very concerned about the health of their oral cavity.

Other psychological concepts which have been explored in relation to oral disorders are self-esteem, self-concept and body image. In most societies certain physical traits are highly valued, so much so that physical appearance and the response of others to it can have important implications for psychological well-being. Dental appearance is an important determinant of facial appearance and can, because of this, have a significant influence on body image and satisfaction with self. Conditions which produce obvious disfigurement, such as facial or palatal clefts, are the most likely to produce psychological problems, although for a proportion of the population less severe abnormalities can have similar effects. Dworkin *et al.* (1978) have developed this point of view and provided a theoretical basis for the belief that the face and mouth play a major role in the development of self-concept. In the context of a society in which facial attractiveness is endowed with such meaning, negative self-concept becomes a major impediment to social and psychological well-being. In a minority of cases, this can become a severe problem. Some patients are so obsessed with the appearance of their teeth and mouth, a condition referred to as dysmorphophobia, that they can be considered to be candidates for psychotherapy.

A number of studies have provided evidence that the appearance of the teeth and mouth is an important issue for many people. Among the teenagers studied by Linn (1976), maintaining or improving appearance was the most common reason cited for taking care of the teeth and gingivae. Among this group, broken or lost permanent teeth, discoloured teeth and teeth that were poorly aligned were major causes of concern. Such concerns are not confined to the young: other age groups, such as people of working age and the elderly, also report being dissatisfied with the appearance of their teeth or dentures (Cushing *et al.* 1986, Locker *et al.* 1987).

Studies that have used measures of self-concept or self-image have also been able to document the effects on self-esteem of oral or facial conditions (Oulette 1978, Klima and McIver 1979). Scores on standardized scales suggest that those with facial deformity or gross malocclusion are lacking in self-confidence and socially withdrawn. However, these effects are not inevitable. Studies of teenagers with facial clefts suggest that they are dependent upon the individual's attitude to and acceptance of their deformity (Starr 1978). One of the few studies which has examined this issue with respect to less severe oral conditions has been reported by Berkey *et al.* (1985). They found that the more mundane dental problems had a negative impact on the self-esteem of elderly people, although the relationship was much stronger for those who retained their own teeth. They suggest that the preservation of the natural dentition is an important psychological concern for many older people who become despondent when the remaining teeth begin to deteriorate markedly. Once all the teeth have been lost, however, the elderly gradually adjust psychologically to this less-than-ideal situation.

Handicap

People with chronic medical conditions, physical disabilities, or other visible abnormalities are frequently denied access to many of the sources of gratification and satisfaction that life in modern societies offers. This denial is largely the product of the deliberate or unwitting responses of others towards those who do not meet conventional standards of appearance or performance. For example, those who are confined to wheelchairs are often unable to take advantage of recreational facilities simply because the buildings in which they are located are not accessible to wheelchairs, and people with fluctuating and variable conditions such as rheumatoid arthritis or mutiple sclerosis are often unable to fulfill their career potential because of frequent absences from work during acute episodes of their condition. Where these conditions are clearly visible, these problems may be compounded by the deliberate exclusion of the person concerned. As a result of these experiences, people with disabling disorders are frequently disadvantaged and do not enjoy the opportunities or material rewards available to the non-disabled.

It should come as no surprise that these problems are encountered by those with facial deformity or the more exaggerated forms of malocclusion. Surprisingly, such handicaps can be experienced even by people with the more common oral conditions. These conditions, like epilepsy, obesity and deafness, can be socially stigmatizing. The word 'stigma' refers to any physical or behavioural attribute which is negatively valued and leads a person to be regarded as unacceptable or inferior. This is partly a product of the condition itself and partly a product of the unjustified imputation of other negative characteristics to the person concerned. In Britain in the 1950s it was rare for children to wear glasses. Those who did were either objects of pity or ridicule, and they were often believed to be stupid. Similarly, in the 1980s people who are obese are frequently regarded as moral degenerates.

These responses are, however, historically and culturally variable. In some societies, people with epilepsy are shunned or excluded, while in others they are believed to possess special powers and accorded high social status. Variation also exists in the value attached to less significant attributes. In Nigeria, for example, it is not uncommon for people to ask their dentist to create a mid-line diastema, whereas in countries such as the UK or the US it is more likely to be viewed as an unfortunate or undesirable trait.

The discrimination that affects those with observable oral conditions may be overt and deliberate or covert and largely unintended. Nevertheless, it can affect either the quality of the person's daily life or even their long-term life chances. An example of the former would be the teasing and harassment suffered by children with abnormal dental features. In one study (Shaw *et al.* 1980a) 66 per cent of 9- to 13-year-olds reported being teased about some physical characteristic or other, dental appearance being the fourth most common feature singled out for ridicule or abuse. One tenth of this group reported being teased at least once a week about prominent incisors, anterior crowding or other aspects of their dentition. Negative comments about the teeth proved more likely to have an impact on a child than comments about any other physical feature: 60 per cent of those who were the recipients of such comments were hurt or upset by them. Perhaps because the appearance of the face and mouth are highly salient in the formation of a social identity, children who were ridiculed because of their teeth were more than twice as likely than other children to report more generalized verbal or physical intimidation or being victimized by their peers. Shaw *et al.* also emphasize that children judged to be introverted by their teachers more frequently complained about this more general form of harassment.

Evidence of the more subtle form of discrimination mentioned above is to be found in a body of research which has assessed the effect of attractiveness on the social relationships of children and adults. Since the appearance of the face and mouth influences judgements about facial attractiveness, they play a role in the attainment of social and occupational goals. A number of studies have found that teachers rate the behaviour and personality of attractive children more highly and expect them to achieve more academically than their less attractive contemporaries. Such expectations are also shared by parents, who predict greater personal and social success for their attractive children. These expectations about academic performance persist even when the attractive and unattractive children involved have equivalent IQs. Such expectations appear to become a self-fulfilling prophecy, for there are studies which show that unattractive children have lower educational achievements and are less socially skilled. Shaw *et al.* (1980b) take this to be evidence of labelling theory, a sociological approach which explains deviance in terms of a causal relationship between social feedback, self-image and behaviour.

Physical attractiveness can also have an impact on the opportunities of adults. Several studies have shown that fake résumés accompanied by a photograph of an attractive individual are rated more highly by managers than identical résumés accompanied by a photograph of an unattractive individual. Other studies have shown that attractive employees are perceived to be more competent by employers. In a study by Jenny and Proshek (1986), an attractive dentition was judged to be important for occupations considered to be highly prestigious. Other evidence of the effects of oral conditions on long-term life chances comes from a study of people with facial defects resulting from congenital clefts. When compared with a control group, such individuals were more likely to remain single, marry later in life, if they did marry, and remain childless.

The economic impact of oral disorders

The studies reviewed above provide evidence of the impact of oral disorders on the individual. Their impact on the community as a whole is best assessed in terms of their direct and indirect economic costs. The direct costs of oral disorders refer to the amount of money spent by governments, insurance companies and individuals on the prevention and treatment of dental disease. While some economists include only money spent on services provided by professional and para-professional staff, others include the costs of oral health care products such as toothpastes and toothbrushes. Although the concept of direct costs is a relatively simple one, such costs are not easy to measure, largely because of a lack of comprehensive data. This is especially so with respect to dental care systems which are mixed in terms of public and private funding. In Canada, for example, estimates of direct costs must be based on income tax returns filed by dentists, adjusted to take account of the costs of services provided by the provinces, or on reports of personal expenditures obtained in national family expenditure surveys. Both sources omit some direct costs and estimates based on these sources underestimate total expenditure (Leake 1984).

International comparisons of the direct costs of dental care have been made and indicate that expenditures on dental treatments are considerable, absorbing between five and ten per cent of total health care expenditures and from one third to one half of a per cent of Gross National Product. In Canada, the amount spent on dental care during 1980 was 1.3 billion Canadian dollars, representing 0.44 per cent of GNP, 5.8 per cent of total health care costs and 47.4 per cent of out-of-pocket health care costs. The per capita expenditure was $53.51 in 1980, up from $6.12 in 1960. After adjusting for inflation, this is equivalent to an increase of 300 per cent (Leake 1984).

The indirect costs of dental disorders are even more difficult to estimate, the most straightforward method being estimates based on the value of lost productivity. Even this is not a simple matter and it is not surprising that no monetary value has so far been placed on days of work lost due to dental and oral disease. However, given what we know about the direct costs of dental care and the human costs of oral conditions in terms of their social and psychological effects, hard data on indirect economic costs are not necessary in order to demonstrate the significance of these disorders for individuals and the community.

7

Illness behaviour: need and demand for dental care

The discrepancy between the need and the demand for dental care has been a long-standing concern of policy makers and health care practitioners. Policy makers want to know whether services are reaching those in need and how services might be modified in order to promote their use by those in need. Practitioners, however, are more likely to be concerned with the 'inappropriate' use of services. For example, a study of British general medical practitioners found that 25 per cent felt that more than half the patients they saw presented with clinically trivial conditions that did not warrant professional intervention (Cartwright and Anderson 1981). At the same time, doctors are also concerned about delays in seeking treatment. Many of those with serious or potentially serious conditions do not present for professional attention until an advanced stage when therapy is likely to be more difficult, more expensive or less effective. This delay can have tragic results. A study of infant deaths in the first year of life found that 30 per cent were preventable; they were caused by treatable respiratory or gastrointestinal infections which were not presented until it was too late for the condition to be resolved (Palmer *et al.* 1980). Similarly, potentially catastrophic delays have also been observed in people with cancer. In one study 40 per cent of women referred to a hospital clinic for the investigation of breast symptoms had waited more than four weeks between first noticing symptoms and consulting their doctor (Nichols *et al.* 1981). Comparable delays also occur with respect to dental pain.

Many dentists, however, would be more concerned that their patients do not have regular check-ups but only visit when they have pain or other trouble. The rationale underlying these preventive visits is to deal with conditions such as calculus deposits before they have caused disease or to detect disease at the earliest stage possible and treat it with only limited interventions. The 1978 Survey of Adult Dental Health (Todd *et al.* 1982) reported that only 43 per cent of the UK population attended regularly for check-ups, 14 per cent went for an occasional check-up and 43 per cent only went to a dentist when they had problems with their teeth or gums. Stimulating demand from this last group may become even more important if dentists' concerns about 'busyness' continue. The overriding concern of all health professionals, however, is that effective treatment of physical and oral conditions always depends upon the patient's initiative in seeking diagnosis and treatment. Understanding treatment-seeking and utilization behaviour is necessary in order to promote effective and efficient care.

The clinical iceberg

The gap between the need for medical and dental care and the utilization of professional services has been referred to as the 'clinical iceberg' (Last 1963). Simply put, this means that health care professionals only see the tip of the iceberg with respect to the volume of illness in the community. Early health surveys undertaken during the 1950s and 1960s found that nearly everyone studied had experienced one or more symptoms but relatively few had received medical attention. Ninety-five per cent of the 3153 respondents interviewed by Wadsworth *et al.* (1971) reported one or more physical complaints in the two weeks prior to interview, but only 21 per cent had sought professional advice. The remainder used non-prescribed medications to treat these complaints or did nothing at all.

Subsequent studies used health diaries to collect data and were able to provide estimates of the proportion of symptom episodes which did and did not receive professional attention. A symptom episode is defined as the presence of a given symptom on one or more consecutive days. This means that pain on two days separated by a pain-free day would count as two episodes. Studies of women aged 20 to 44 years and 16 to 44 years have been undertaken by Banks *et al.* (1975) and Scambler *et al.* (1981). Some of their results are summarized in Table 7.1. In the former, only one in thirty-seven of the episodes recorded in the health diaries were

Table 7.1 Symptom episodes and medical consultations recorded in health diaries

	Ratio symptom episodes to consultations	
	Banks *et al.* (1975)	Scambler *et al.* (1981)
Headache	184:1	60:1
Changes in energy, tiredness	456:1	—
Nerves, depression, irritability	46:1	74:1
Aches or pains in joints, muscles, legs or arms	49:1*	18:1
Menstrual problems	20:1	10:1
Stomach ache or pain	29:1	11:1
Backache	52:1	38:1
Sore throat	18:1	9:1
Pain in chest	14:1	—
Sleeplessness	—	31:1
Totals	37:1	18:1

* Pain in lower limb only
Source: Banks *et al.* (1975), Scambler *et al.* (1981)

made known to a doctor and in the latter only one in eighteen gave rise to a consultation. Even when pain was involved the ratio still stood at less than one in ten.

One explanation for this discrepancy is that most of the symptoms recorded were minor and did not warrant medical attention. This is certainly the case for a proportion of these symptoms. However, studies involving clinical examinations have shown that many conditions severe enough to need treatment are not made known to a doctor. Epsom (1969) gave a comprehensive medical examination to 3000 persons aged 16 to 60 years, 22 per cent of whom were referred to their family doctor for further investigation and treatment of conditions not previously diagnosed and 5 per cent were eventually referred to hospital or specialist out-patient clinics. An even higher proportion of untreated severe conditions were found in a study of 200 persons aged 65 or over. A third of those with heart disease, a quarter of those with bronchitis and nine out of ten with depression were not receiving treatment (Williamson 1964).

In all population-based surveys of dental health, substantial proportions of those examined are found to need treatment for one or more conditions. For example, the National Health and

Nutrition Examination Survey of 1971–4 estimated that 65 per cent of the US adult population needed dental treatment of one type or another. Just over 40 per cent required restorations and 5 per cent extractions (Striffler 1983). Among the dentate adults examined during the 1978 survey of adults in the UK, 48 per cent of those who went to a dentist regularly had one or more decayed teeth and 57 per cent of those who went infrequently needed treatment for decay. Calculus, gingivitis and periodontal disease were found in 91 per cent, and 27 per cent needed partial dentures (Todd *et al.* 1982). A more recent Canadian study of persons aged 50 years and over found high levels of treatment need; 95 per cent of the dentate and 66 per cent of the edentulous required one or more dental services (Locker *et al.* 1987).

One explanation of these high levels of unmet need is that diseases like caries and periodontitis are frequently asymptomatic and invisible to the untrained eye. Consequently, those affected may be unaware of the presence of disease and the need for treatment. Some support for this is found in the data presented by Todd *et al.* (1982). They found that 60 per cent of adults with one to five decayed teeth and 26 per cent of those with 6 or more decayed teeth were unaware of the presence of decay. However, the iceberg persists when we look at symptoms rather than disease. In the survey of oral and facial pain described in Chapter 6, 40 per cent of respondents reported one or more of nine pain symptoms in the four weeks preceding completion of the questionnaire. Of these, only 44 per cent had sought professional attention. It was somewhat of a surprise to find that there was no significant association between the severity of the pain and treatment seeking. Almost 48 per cent of those with severe pain had not been to the dentist. This analysis was repeated for those reporting toothache, and essentially the same results emerged: a substantial proportion of those in severe pain had not sought treatment — see Table 7.2 (Locker 1988). Similar observations were made by Hannay (1980), who asked a random sample of patients registered with a health centre to complete a symptom questionnaire, to state the severity of the pain or disability associated with each symptom recorded, and evaluate its seriousness. Twenty-six per cent of those reporting severe symptoms had not been to the doctor, while 11 per cent of those with symptoms which did not cause pain or disability and which were not perceived as serious had consulted their general practitioner. Table 7.3 gives the results of another study which obtained data on the proportion of people with various

Table 7.2 Oral and facial pain: percentage seeking professional attention by severity of the pain

	All oral and facial pain*	Toothache
Mild	41.0	50.0
Moderately severe	47.1	42.8
Severe	52.2	61.5

* Responding to one or more of nine pain items
Source: Locker 1988

Table 7.3 Percentage of persons with various dental conditions who made dental visits

Condition	% making visit
Toothache	75
Sore or bleeding gums	45
Loss of permanent tooth	61
Pain in tooth when drinking hot and cold fluids	54
Calculus or stains on teeth	57
Crooked teeth	32

Source: Anderson and Newman 1973

oral conditions who sought dental treatment. These data indicate that the mere presence of disease or symptoms, irrespective of their severity, is not sufficient to stimulate the seeking of professional care; social, psychological and organizational factors are involved in the process which ends with a consultation.

The gap between the need for and use of health services has two important implications. First, a significant proportion of the population are subject to pain, discomfort or other problems caused by conditions which would respond to treatment. Unmet need has a direct impact on the quality of life of the community. Second, it suggests that treated cases are not representative of sufferers as a whole and that knowledge of disorders obtained by the study of such cases is likely to be biased. A clear example of this is the relationship between sex and temporomandibular disorders (TMD). Early studies based on those who sought treatment characterized the condition as one which predominantly affected women. Subsequently, population-based studies showed that the sex distribution of the condition was not the same as the sex distribution of cases with men and women affected to almost the same degree (Locker and Slade 1988).

Definitions of need and demand

A number of definitions of need and demand have been developed over the last few years. Those offered by Spencer (1980) will suffice here. *Normative* need refers to the need for a service or services as determined by a professional or other expert, *perceived* need is the need for care as defined by the patient, *demand* arises out of the desire or attempt by the public to seek professional care, and *utilization* represents the actual use of services. In practice, little real distinction is drawn between demand and utilization and they are often taken to mean the same thing. Clearly, normative and perceived need may differ, perceived need may not give rise to demand, and the demand may not be translated into utilization. It is often the case that patients are satisfied with dentures that have been judged by a professional to be clinically unsatisfactory in terms of retention and fit. This difference of opinion arises because patients are able to adapt to and chew adequately with dentures considered unacceptable according to the criteria applied by the professional.

The most common way of estimating the dental health care needs of a population is by the use of dental surveys. Here, need may be assessed in terms of numbers of people, numbers of procedures, hours of manpower, or costs. In addition, need may be based on assessments of untreated disease, the presence of discomfort, or the disability that arises out of disease. A number of indices have been developed for translating data on disease prevalence into assessments of the volume and type of services required.

Utilization is measured by social surveys and analyses of patient records. The former provide data on the characteristics of utilizers and non-utilizers and give estimates of the proportion using the service in a given time period and the mean number of visits in that period. Data on actual services consumed and the cost of those services are less easy to obtain due to a lack of knowledge on the part of respondents or failures in recall. Such data can be gathered from patient records but no information is obtained which would allow users and non-users to be compared.

Studies of the need–demand problem fall into one of two types. The first consists of studies of utilization of medical and dental care. These studies are largely concerned with who uses health services and why. In answering this question data have been collected on the characteristics of individuals and the characteristics of services, particularly those which are believed to promote or hinder utilization. The second consists of studies of health and illness behaviour. These have attempted to understand the response to the signs, symptoms, or threat of disease and the role played by social and psychological factors in this process.

The utilization of dental care

Estimates of the proportion of the population using dental services suggest a substantial increase over the past forty to fifty years. In 1930, 21 per cent of the US population had made at least one visit to the dentist in the previous year and by 1979 this had risen to 55 per cent. UK data show the same trend; from 18 per cent in 1949 to 49 per cent in 1978. Canadian studies indicate that utilization rates rose from 15 per cent in 1950–51 to about 50 per cent in 1978–9. The growth of public and private insurance schemes, the growth in the number of dentists, rising incomes and educational standards, and a trend towards healthier lifestyles are some of the factors which have influenced the volume and pattern of dental care utilization. Even so, major inequalities in use exist between socioeconomic groups and different geographic regions of these countries.

Many of the studies on which our understanding of utilization is based were undertaken between 1964 and 1974 (Gift 1984). A great deal of effort was devoted to describing the characteristics of those who did and did not use services and to identifying barriers which prevented predominantly low-income groups from receiving treatment when in need. Interest in utilization declined during the late 1970s and 1980s when cost containment emerged as the dominant policy issue. Nevertheless, the case can be made that understanding utilization and identifying barriers to care is even more important during a time of restraint on health care spending. Cost containment programmes and the development of alternative delivery systems may make access to care more difficult for the poor or other disadvantaged groups.

McKinlay (1972) has identified six different groups of factors which have been included in studies of utilization and which are believed to be important in seeking dental and medical care. These are: *socio-demographic* factors such as age, sex and race; *economic* factors such as income and price of services; *socio-psychological* factors such as motivation, perception and learning; *socio-cultural* factors such as the values, beliefs and lifestyles of cultural or sub-cultural groups; *geographic* factors such as the proximity of services and travelling time to health care facilities; and *organizational* factors such as type of delivery system and population–practitioner ratios. Anderson and Newman (1973) have further classified these into three broad types: predisposing factors, enabling factors, and factors related to need. The first represents a person's propensity to use services, the second includes barriers or aids which limit or promote access to services and the third refers to objective and subjectively perceived needs for health care.

Over the period reviewed above, the demographic profile of the users of dental services has remained fairly stable. Women, older children and young adults, high income earners, the more highly educated, and urban residents are the greatest users of dental care. One of the most powerful of these explanatory factors is age. Most studies show that the relationship between utilization and age takes the form of an inverted U-shaped curve, with the very young and the old having very low rates of use. Low utilization by the elderly reflects the fact that the proportion without natural teeth is highest in this section of the population. If only the dentate are considered, then the gap between the young and the old remains but it is not nearly so pronounced. It is anticipated that demographic and other changes, particularly changes in needs and attitudes among the elderly population, will eliminate much of the relationship between age and use of dental services.

When so many factors are actually or potentially related to the use of dental care it is important to be able to assess the relative and independent significance of each of these factors. The development of multivariate statistical techniques has facilitated this exercise. Summarizing the results of such studies can be difficult since they use different measures of utilization as their dependent variable and include different numbers and types of independent or predictor variables.

In a study confined to the Canadian province of Ontario, Bullen (1982) found that the most important variable which predicted the actual number of visits to a dentist during the years 1979–80 was the retention of natural teeth. When an analysis was undertaken for the dentate only, family income proved to be the most important predictor. For the population as a whole, the factors which determined dental care utilization were dental status, family income, the local dentist–population ratio, age, insurance coverage, occupation, and community size. A study using a national sample of the Canadian population found that the most important factors in order of their predictive power were age, education, dentist–population ratios, a perceived dental problem, sex, family income, family size, marital status, and employment status (Manga and Charette 1986). Even though the dependent variable in this study was one or more visits during the previous year, there are broad similarities between these provincial and national surveys.

One problem with these studies is that they do not include variables concerning attitudes and beliefs. These are important, since positive attitudes will increase the propensity to seek care. In studies of elderly populations Kiyak (1984) found that the addition of subjective variables such as perceived importance of dental health, beliefs about dental health, and perceived need for dental care were not only important in their own right, but improved the overall predictive power of statistical models of utilization behaviour.

It should be recognized, however, that while some variables may be of statistical importance, they may be unimportant from a policy perspective. Where the aim is to improve access to dental care, the most significant variables are those that can be most easily manipulated by cost-effective policy initiatives. The most common initiatives are health education and the removal or reduction of economic barriers by the provision of free care, or the development of public and/or private dental health insurance schemes (see Chapter 14).

The study of health and illness behaviour

Kasl and Cobb (1966) defined health behaviour as any activity undertaken by individuals who see themselves as healthy for the purpose of preventing disease or detecting it at an asymptomatic stage. In the context of dentistry this would include brushing and flossing the teeth, avoiding high sugar foods and visiting the dentist at regular intervals for check-ups. Illness behaviour they defined as any activity undertaken by individuals who perceive themselves as having a health problem for the purpose of defining their state of health and discovering and undertaking an appropriate remedy. The study of illness behaviour attempts to answer the question, in the presence of signs and symptoms, what will an individual do and why? This may, but does not necessarily involve, seeking professional care.

An early contribution to the understanding of health behaviour is to be found in the Health Belief Model (HBM) (Rosenstock 1966). This model, which is reviewed further in Chapter 11, suggests that health behaviour is a function of a set of interacting beliefs. In order to be motivated to take action to avoid illness, an individual must be in a state of readiness to take action and believe that the action would have positive outcomes. In order to be ready to act, the individual would need to feel susceptible to the disease in question and to believe that it would have a significant impact on some aspect of his or her life. Beliefs about the benefits of action also involve beliefs about barriers to action such as time, cost, inconvenience and pain. In order to enhance its rather limited explanatory power, this simple model was subsequently extended to include cues and modifying factors. Cues consist of specific events, such as the perception of symptoms or the receipt of a reminder card, which act as a stimulus to action. Modifying factors consist of demographic variables (such as age, sex and race), socio-psychological variables (personality, peer, and reference group pressures) and structural variables (such as knowledge and prior experience of the disease). All of these condition the perception of susceptibility and seriousness, and the perception of the benefits of health-related behaviour. As will be described in Chapter 11, the model has not performed that well when subject to empirical testing. It has also been used to predict illness behaviour and the likelihood that an individual will comply with a therapeutic regimen prescribed by a health professional (Becker 1977). Again, although specific factors included in the model are associated with these health-related behaviours, overall it explains little in the way of observed variation in behaviour.

The Anderson and Newman model of health service utilization described above includes variables of many types. In considering the response to symptoms, however, Mechanic (1968) lays greater emphasis on the character of the symptoms themselves. He has identified the following ten variables to be important in the seeking of professional advice:

1 the visibility, recognizability, and perceptual salience of the symptoms;

2 the perceived seriousness of the symptoms;

3 the extent to which symptoms disrupt work, family, and other social activities;

4 the frequency of the appearance of symptoms and their persistence or frequency of recurrence;

5 the tolerance thresholds of others who are exposed to the symptoms;

6 the knowledge, cultural assumptions and understanding of the person and relevant others;

7 other needs or practical matters competing with the illness response;

8 competing possible interpretations which can be assigned to symptoms once recognized;

9 emotional barriers in the form of fear and anxiety which influence the choice of actions to deal with the problem; and

10 the availability, physical proximity, and the financial and/or emotional costs of taking various courses of action.

Evidence of the relevance of some of the factors comes from the study of oral and facial pain described above. Although the severity of the pain was not associated with seeing a dentist, a number of variables describing the character and impact of the symptoms were. Treatment-seeking was related to the number of pain symptoms reported, the mean number of days on which pain was experienced, and past pain experience assessed in terms of the frequency of pain episodes in the past year. Those who reported that pain had an impact on daily living were also more likely to have sought professional advice. The most important impact was sleep disturbance; 63 per cent of those who had been kept awake at night had seen a dentist.

These approaches to health and illness behaviour are often termed 'individualistic' approaches. This means they attempt to explain variations in behaviour primarily in terms of the characteristics of individuals. Other approaches have been termed 'collectivist'; that is, they explain these variations in terms of the characteristics of the social groups to which the individual belongs. As Freidson has argued:

> In the process of imputing meaning to his experience the individual sufferer does not invent the meanings himself but rather uses the meanings and interpretations that his social

> life has provided him. Thus, one can predict the behaviour of a collection of individuals without reference to their individual characteristics, by referring solely to the context of the social life in which they participate. (Freidson 1970: 288–9)

The culture within which an individual has been raised provides the individual with a body of knowledge about health and illness and about the kind of actions to take when some departure from normal functioning is observed. These meanings and prescriptions for action may or may not be congruent with those of professional providers. In fact, differences may be observed between ethnic groups and also between members of different socioeconomic groups. Low-income groups, for example, may not attach the same meaning and significance to symptoms such as pain or bleeding gums as a professional. In some instances these may be seen as part of the normal pattern of everyday life and not give rise to much concern, let alone a professional consultation.

However, once some state of departure from normal functioning is recognized, Freidson claims that the type of help sought is influenced by a 'lay referral system'. That is, people in the individual's social network, such as family members or friends, are consulted and the decision about an appropriate means of dealing with the problem decided jointly. Two characteristics of this lay referral system are of importance in determining whether doing nothing, using a 'folk' remedy or proprietary medicine, or arranging a professional consultation is the action of choice. The first is the gap between the lay culture in question and the beliefs and attitudes of health care professionals. The second is the size and degree of cohesiveness of the group and the extent to which it is open to outside influences. Where the culture of the lay referral system is markedly different from that of professionals, is extended and highly cohesive, then rates of utilization of health services as a means of dealing with health-related problems will be low. Studies of the use of preventive services and general practitioner services have shown that the size and composition of a person's social network and the number and types of individuals consulted, whether lay or kin, influence the use of services (McKinlay 1973, Scambler *et al.* 1981).

Illness behaviour as a decision-making process

One way of organizing the results of studies of utilization and of research generated by individualistic and collectivistic approaches to illness behaviour is to view the response to symptoms and the actions involved in that response as a decision-making process. This process is implied in an early definition of the field offered by Mechanic (1968: 19): 'By illness behaviour we mean the way symptoms are perceived, evaluated and acted upon by a person who recognises some pain, discomfort or other signs of organic malfunction.'

The time period over which this decision-making process takes place and its outcome in the form of health-related behaviours are determined by the nature of the event that triggers the process and the nature of the situation within which it occurs. For example, some symptoms may be so dramatic that they are immediately recognized as events requiring medical attention. Acute pain, a sudden loss of blood, or total collapse would fall into this category. Most symptoms, however, are ambiguous and it may not be clear whether they represent normal variation in the structure and functioning of the body, or whether they indicate some potentially serious disorder. The extent to which the problem disrupts daily life may be a factor taken into account in this initial decision. Other situational factors, termed 'triggers' by Zola (1973), may also play a role. Even if these symptoms are interpreted as an indication of illness, the individual must still decide whether or not it is sufficiently serious to warrant professional attention. It is during the making of these judgements that culturally derived knowledge about health and illness, the influence of others, and past experience with illness and health care providers have their greatest effect. Past experience with health care may, along with time, money, and fear, create a barrier to formal health care. Many are reluctant to seek professional advice for fear of criticism that they have bothered a busy health care provider with routine complaints that could be managed at home.

Clearly, the decision-making processes which result in the use of a professional service are complex, fluid, and difficult to pin down. This should indicate that human behaviour with respect to health cannot be explained simply and easily by reference to one or more variables that characterize the services themselves or the people who do or do not use them. These variables are related to service use but ultimately explain very little. They do, however, offer guidelines as to what kind of interventions may be necessary to stimulate a greater or lesser resort to professional attention.

The 'appropriate' use of professional health care

One of the major contributions of the work on health and illness behaviour is that it can assist professionals to make sense of the apparently 'irrational' behaviour of patients. The failure to use obviously beneficial preventive services or the delay in seeking treatment for acute pain can seem puzzling to the provider of a service who believes in its effectiveness and desirability. It is clear that many providers judge patient behaviour in terms of the clinical significance of the problems that present or in terms of scientifically based estimates of the health risks associated with certain types of lifestyle. Patients, however, use a different system of knowledge to make such judgements about significance and risk. An appreciation of the differing cultural contexts in which these judgements are made and the specific events which stimulate the seeking of care can be of value in managing both the patient and the presenting problem. A number of authors have suggested that questioning the patient about the timing of a consultation — why now? — provides useful information about the patient's view of the problem and their particular concerns with respect to it. It may reveal worries and anxieties or other issues that need to be dealt with in the process of providing care (see Chapter 8). It will also forestall any overt or implied criticism of the patient's conduct which can seriously affect patient satisfaction with their health care provider.

Accepting that the process of seeking preventive and treatment services is a complex one does not necessarily mean that interventions to change levels of use or close the gap between need and demand cannot be identified. Strategies to change levels or patterns of use require only that important factors and their relative significance are known. In terms of dental care there are three distinct groups of under-utilizers who may be the targets for such intervention. These are: (1) *effective utilizers*, who desire treatment and are able to obtain it; (2) *potential utilizers*, who desire treatment but are prevented from obtaining it by one or more barriers; and (3) true *under-utilizers*, who need treatment but do not perceive or desire it (Douglass and Cole 1979). These would include those who only used services on an emergency basis.

Effective utilizers are under-utilizers to the extent that they may seek treatment but not preventive services. Any change with respect to this group would involve reducing the need for treatment by an emphasis on oral self-care and early diagnosis. In the case of potential utilizers, the problem is one of removing economic or organizational barriers which limit access to care. In the case of the true under-utilizers, changing service use would require substantial changes in both motivation and behaviour.

The types of interventions that are likely to be successful will vary according to the weight attached to the kinds of variables investigated in utilization studies. If knowledge, beliefs, and attitudes are believed to be the problem, then some kind of educational programme specifically targeted at under-utilizing groups is required. If more weight is attached to the role of fear in preventing visits to the dentist, then training dentists in the control of pain and anxiety may have an effect. If economic or organizational barriers are believed to be significant, then providing care free, or at a reduced charge, or changing the structure of services would be the policy option of choice. All of these attempt to manipulate the way the individual perceives the costs and benefits of professional care. Aspects of these strategies are addressed in later chapters.

8
Dentist–patient communication

A dentist, like all other health professionals, must develop a variety of skills in order to provide safe and effective patient care. In dental education most emphasis is usually placed upon *clinical* and *technical* skills. These include the ability to recognize the signs and symptoms of disease, interpret the results of radiographic or other diagnostic tests, arrive at a competent diagnosis and undertake the often complex manual procedures involved in the provision of surgical, restorative and prosthodontic treatment. Traditionally, less significance has been attached to the development of *scientific* skills, the ability to evaluate knowledge about the distribution, causes, and treatment of disease, and *interpersonal* skills, the ability to develop a satisfactory relationship with patients, manage patient behaviour, and provide for the social and psychological needs of patients.

Increasingly, it has been recognized that the interpersonal aspects of health care, particularly the practitioner–patient relationship, are as essential to the treatment of patients and their health problems as the drugs or other therapies that are prescribed. Clearly, communication between practitioner and patient is important, for it provides the foundation for diagnosis and treatment. The professional must be able to elicit information from the patient, even though the patient may have some difficulty in describing their symptoms or revealing their problem, and must, in turn, be adept at conveying information to the patient about the nature of his or her problem and the treatment necessary to deal with it. However, the significance of the practitioner–patient relationship goes beyond this, for the relationship itself has a powerful therapeutic effect. This is akin to the placebo effect observed in relation to the prescribing and taking of drugs. A failure to develop a satisfactory relationship with a patient means that this therapeutic benefit is not obtained.

Judging by the volume and scope of research conducted to date, the doctor–patient relationship has been accorded greater significance than the relationship between dentist and patient. Reviews of the literature on the dentist–patient relationship by Linn (1971) and Ayer and Corah (1984) suggest that only a narrow range of issues have been examined. Much of the research reported in the literature has been concerned with behavioural problems, especially with respect to children, and psychological problems, such as anxiety, which impede the provision of dental treatment (see Chapters 9 and 10). This reflects a tendency to view dental care as primarily a set of technical procedures performed *on* a patient with dental disease. Given the current emphasis on patient education, motivation and preventive oral health behaviours, the perspective needs to be broadened considerably to encompass dentist–patient interaction and its positive and negative outcomes.

Because of the narrowness of the approach to the dentist–patient relationship, it is necessary to draw on the literature covering the doctor–patient relationship in order to develop the themes mentioned above. Much of this work is directly applicable to dentistry and, along with the literature on the other healing professions, can be used to identify the salient features of the practitioner–patient relationship and its therapeutic benefits.

Types of doctor–patient relationship

Ayer and Corah (1984) believe that one of the major limitations of the research on dentists and patients is its general failure to recognize that there are many types of dentist–patient relationships. Szasz and Hollender (1956), in an early contribution to the field, described three relationships which characterize consultations between doctors and patients. Which of these is evident in any particular consultation will vary according to the patient's condition and the nature of the treatment offered.

The first type of relationship, the 'activity–passivity' model, is one in which the doctor assumes complete responsibility for the patient's treatment. The most extreme form of this relationship exists when the patient is in a state whereby he or she cannot respond to the doctor, such as a coma, state of collapse, or when under general anaesthetic. In a less extreme form, this model is characteristic of many dentist–patient encounters. Many dental consultations involve, at least for much of the time, the patient lying passively in the chair while the dentist undertakes some restorative or other procedure. Evidence, admittedly somewhat dated now, suggests that patients are similarly passive even when not confined to the chair. Rayner (1970) observed that verbal interactions between dentists and patients were minimal and Linn (1974) observed that patients rarely initiated conversation with the dentist, with two thirds of patients reporting that they never asked anyone in the dental office for information or advice. They assumed that the dentist would tell them what they needed to know.

The second type of relationship, the 'guidance–cooperation' model, is probably the most common and is one in which the doctor instructs the patient on what needs to be done about the presenting complaint and the patient cooperates by following this advice. However, the relationship described as 'mutual participation' is becoming more common, largely because of the increased prevalence of chronic disease and the need for preventive health behaviours. A good example is to be found in dental health education. Here, the dentist provides the patient with the necessary knowledge and skills and the patient then takes responsibility for improving and maintaining his or her oral hygiene. In this model, the professional helps patients to help themselves.

Although the encounters between doctors and patients are constrained by the patient's condition and the nature of the treatment offered, the relationship between them is highly variable. It may change over the course of the patient's treatment or during the course of a single consultation. The relationship is also subject to modification by the patient and the practitioner. However, given that the practitioner is generally in control of the consultation it is his or her preferences and perceptions of the patient which will ultimately determine its form.

Consensus and conflict in patient–practitioner relationships

The typology presented by Szasz and Hollender is an example of what is usually termed the 'consensus' approach to the doctor–patient relationship. This approach has its origins in an analysis of the functions of medical practice undertaken by Parsons in the early 1950s (Parsons 1951). Parsons, a sociologist, believed that medicine performs an essential function for society: it restores the sick to health and enables the individual concerned to resume their usual work and family roles.

This process of restoring a sick individual to health is facilitated by the respective roles of doctor and patient, both of which carry rights and obligations. The patient is granted exemption from some or all of the usual social responsibilities, but is obliged to seek professional help and cooperate fully in the process of getting well. In turn, the doctor is granted access to the patient's body, accorded a position of authority in relation to the patient, and allowed considerable autonomy in terms of professional practice. However, the doctor is obliged to abide by rules of professional conduct, act in the best interests of the patient, and to proceed in an objective, scientific manner.

Parsons saw the roles of doctor and patient as complementary and the doctor–patient relationship characterized by harmony and agreement over the aims and objectives of the consultation. Others, notably Freidson (1970), believe that the doctor–patient relationship is characterized by conflict rather than harmony. This conflict, which rarely surfaces during the actual consultation, originates in the different perspectives of doctor and patient. The doctor views the patient's condition in a detached, scientific manner and evaluates its severity and significance according to clinical criteria. The patient, however, is more personally involved with the illness and assesses its significance in terms of its social and psychological impact and is implications for his or her life as a whole. Moreover, patients have their own, often sophisticated, ideas about the nature and causes of their illness which do not necessarily match the 'scientific' account presented by the doctor. Evidence of such conflicting perspectives comes from studies which show that doctors and patients rate the clinical and social significance of various symptoms quite differently, and from the frequent complaints of doctors that too many of their patients present for treatment with clinically trivial conditions. What the patient may view as a potentially serious symptom worthy of professional attention may be viewed by the doctor as a medically insignificant complaint that could have been managed by the patient at home (see Chapter 7). Detailed accounts of how such conflicts are handled or not handled in the context of a consultation are to be found in Stimson and Webb (1975).

Communication and health care provision

Communication is now regarded by both health professionals and social scientists as a key process in health care provision. It provides the foundation for diagnosis and treatment and is closely associated with therapeutic outcomes. Communication is also important to the patient. Information provided by health professionals is necessary to allow patients to make sense of, to manage and to feel at ease with their health problems. Despite the significance attached to communication, it remains a major area of patient dissatisfaction. Studies of hospital patients, general practice patients, and dental patients conducted between 1960 and 1985 all show that complaints are more frequently expressed about the amount and nature of the information that is given than about any other aspect of treatment and care. In a study of general practice in the US, patients were asked if they had received enough information about the diagnosis, aetiology, treatment, and prognosis of their condition: only 56 per cent felt they had been fully informed (Kincey *et al.* 1975). In a study in the UK, 23 per cent of patients felt that their doctor was not good at explaining things to them (Cartwight and Anderson 1981). Similar results have been reported with respect to dentistry. Collett (1969) estimated that 25 per cent of patients left a dental practice over a five-year period because of poor dentist–patient communication and Corah (1974) estimated that such loss was as high as 50 per cent. Of some interest, then, are the reasons why communication between health professionals and their patients is less than it ought to be. A number of explanations of poor communication have been offered, each of which contributes to our understanding of the complexities of the practitioner–patient relationship.

Explaining poor communication

The influence of class and status

Poor communication is often attributed to differences in class and status between patients and their professional health care providers. Such differences lead to diffidence on the part of patients and a reluctance to make demands on the professional's time. For example, in a study of patients in hospital, only 45 per cent obtained the information they desired by asking doctors or nurses directly. The rest either waited to be told what they wished to know or received no information at all (Cartwright 1964). However, there were social class differences in the way patients acquired information, with middle-class patients more likely to ask for information than the working class. The observation that people similar to doctors and dentists in terms of social class are more able to communicate effectively with them is supported by a number of studies of general practice, some of which were mentioned in Chapter 3. Working-class patients say less than middle-class patients about their problems, they ask fewer questions, get less information and are offered fewer explanations despite the fact that they wish to know as much as possible about their health.

Doctors and dentists may contribute to these class differences in communication as a result of their perceptions of and assumptions about patients. Frazier *et al.* (1977) found that persons on low incomes placed a high priority on dental care but were perceived by their dentists as placing a low priority on dental health. Further, Weinstein *et al.* (1978) found that patients who were perceived by their dentists to value dental care received better restorative care. It is not unreasonable to suppose that health professionals offer less information to those whom they assume do not share their values with respect to oral health.

Cognitive failure

A second explanation which lays more emphasis on cognitive processes sees poor communication as having its origins in failures in comprehension, interpretation, and memory. Even when professionals make special efforts to communicate more effectively, many patients remain dissatisfied. Ley and Spelman (1976) believe that this is due to certain features of the patient–practitioner relationship which inhibit patients' understanding and retention of information. First, patients are not familiar with the technical language of medicine and may not understand messages which are presented in this technical vocabulary. Second, many patients find consultation with doctors and dentists anxiety-provoking and anxiety has a negative effect on memory. Third, time constraints may mean that, when information is given to the patient, too much is presented too quickly, resulting in a selective recall of what has been told. There is some evidence to support this point of view. Studies by Ley and Spelman and others have shown that patients are often unable to remember more than 50 per cent of the information they were given, even five minutes after the end of the consultation (see Table 8.1).

Table 8.1 Summary of studies of patients forgetting medical information

Investigators	Study	Time between consultation and recall	% forgotten
Ley and Spelman (1965)	47 outpatients	10–80 min	37.2
Ley and Spelman (1967)	(a) 22 outpatients	10–80 min	38.7
	(b) 22 outpatients	10–80 min	40.6
Joyce *et al.*	(a) 30 outpatients	Immediately after consultation	52.0
	(b) 24 outpatients	1 to 4 weeks	54.0
Ley *et al.* (1973)	20 general practice patients	Less than 5 minutes	50.0

Source: Ley (1976)

More recently, researchers have begun to explore the cultural differences between patients and health professionals and their impact on communication. This work takes its cue from the 'conflict of perspectives' identified by Freidson (1970) as an integral feature of the doctor–patient relationship. The problem is not that patients lack knowledge about medical matters but draw on a body of knowledge and belief concerning the causes and course of illness acquired from personal experience or the ideas prevalent in the social groups to which they belong. Patients' presentation of their problem is shaped by these ideas about illness and appropriate forms of treatment, whereas the professional approach to the problem is derived from clinical science. If these lay and medical models of disease and its treatment differ, then the professional may have trouble eliciting the information needed to make a diagnosis, while the patient will have trouble getting the professional to respond to his or her own views and concerns (Boulton *et al.* 1986). To the extent that the 'lay theories' of the patient are not known to or appreciated by the practitioner, communication is likely to be poor. The significance of these lay beliefs in terms of the cognitive outcomes of the consultation has been reported by Tuckett *et al.* (1985). A detailed study of 1302 consultations and patients' responses to them found that patients understood and accepted the doctor's views only when they were consistent with their own lay theories. When the doctor's views were different from their own and when these conflicting opinions were not resolved during the consultation, then patients misinterpreted or rejected elements of what the doctor told them. This happened in 50 per cent of the consultations observed. Patients with minimal education and those from minority backgrounds were the most likely to misunderstand or reject the doctor's comments, largely because they drew on alternative views of medical matters which had authority and validity in the social group to which these patients belonged.

Professional attitudes and interviewing styles

While the explanations reviewed above tend to emphasize the role of the patient in poor communication, the final two accounts tend to focus more on the practitioner. The first concerns professional attitudes towards communication and the interviewing styles adopted by professionals in dealing with their clients.

Studies of both dentists and doctors suggest that both types of practitioner regard the education of patients as an important part of their work, although many feel inadequately trained to do it and often find it is difficult to accomplish because of a lack of time. However, not all practitioners view the transmission of information to patients in this way. Comarroff (1976) interviewed general medical practitioners and found that some deliberately gave as little information as possible to their patients. Patients who asked for information were given only limited explanations, while those who did not ask were given none. These doctors had a somewhat paternalistic view of their patients and withheld information on the grounds that it only caused the patient to become worried or anxious. Other doctors saw the communication of information as an integral part of their job and gave their patients as much information as possible in the time available, although they did vary the complexity of the explanations they gave according to their judgements about the patient's ability to understand.

Poor communication may also be an unintended outcome of the interviewing style adopted by the practitioner. This may effectively limit the participation of the patient in the encounter and prevent the patient from raising his or her own particular worries and concerns. In studies of doctor–patient interviews by Plaja and Cohen (1968) and Byrne and Long (1976), the most common style observed was one which is best described as 'bureaucratic-task oriented'. This style involves a simple information-gathering technique, characterized by efficient questioning and limited sensitivity to the patient. The patients of these doctors responded by matter-of-fact collaboration with the doctor's questions and took little initiative in broadening the dialogue. The patient's concerns and feelings were rarely discussed and the doctors tended to be unresponsive to information which was not directly relevant to the medical investigation of the patient's symptoms. This can be contrasted with a 'person-oriented' style of patient management, in which empathy and awareness of the patient's feelings are central to the consultation. In this approach, human concerns are not regarded as an impediment to an efficient consultation, but are treated as an essential component of patient care.

Professional power

This explanation claims that poor communication is a product of the doctor's need to maintain power and professional authority over the patient. Because of their professional status practitioners are almost wholly responsible for the conduct of a consultation. They initiate lines of questioning and control the flow of information back to the patient. The patient is thereby relegated to a relatively subordinate role and there is often little opportunity to influence either the course of the consultation or the diagnostic and treatment decisions flowing from it. The study of 1302 consultations mentioned above found that while three quarters of patients made some attempt to influence the consultation, either by suggesting a diagnosis, requesting further explanation, asking for clarification, or doubting the doctor's interpretation, the manner in which they did so was generally weak and unsuccessful (Boulton *et al.* 1986).

The tight control of a consultation and the limited patient access to information have a number of benefits for a practitioner. At a minimum, they allow the practitioner to limit the length of the consultation by restricting the patient's ability to raise questions. They also allow the practitioner to deal with the ubiquitous issue of uncertainty. *Clinical uncertainty* arises when there is ambiguity over the nature, cause, or prognosis of the patient's condition — an increasingly common occurrence given the prevalence of chronic illness in the population. In these instances a failure to inform patients masks this uncertainty and maintains the patient's belief in the practitioner's competence. *Functional uncertainty* arises with diseases such as cancer, when the diagnosis and prognosis, usually unfavourable, is known. In these cases, the 'bad news' is kept from the patient by subtle communication techniques which maintain the patient's uncertainty about the condition. In this way, doctors are able to avoid the emotional outbursts or negative patient responses which might otherwise follow disclosure of this information.

The benefits of improved communication

Compliance with medical instructions and advice

Compliance refers to the extent to which patients follow instructions and advice given to them by dentists and doctors. Evidence suggests that non-compliance is a major problem in health care. A recent review of research indicated that over 40 per cent of patients fail to take prescribed medications, and over 50 per cent do not follow dietary or other advice. Clearly, this has both economic and therapeutic implications. Initial investigations of non-compliance focused on the patient and attempted, without success, to identify a 'non-cooperative type'. More recently, the problem has been seen to reside in failures in practitioner–patient communication. Support for this point of view has come from Kincey *et al.* (1975), who found that patient satisfaction with the amount of information received during a consultation was associated with compliance with the doctor's advice. Similarly, the extent to which a mother followed advice provided by paediatricians was related to the extent to which the doctors understood the mother's concerns with respect to her child and, most importantly of all, provided sufficient information about the child's disorder (Korsch *et al.* 1969). Where an explanation of the nature and cause of the child's illness was not given, non-compliance increased from 11 per cent to 24 per cent.

More recent studies have also emphasized the significance of the doctor–patient relationship in terms of subsequent compliance. Low compliance tends to be associated with doctors who do not seek the patient's active participation in the interview, are formal or distant in their management of the patient and provide little in the way of feedback. By contrast, patient-centred interviews, in which the views and opinions of the patient are discussed, are associated with much higher levels of compliance (Stewart 1984), most probably because the chances of patients misinterpreting or rejecting the doctor's treatment plan are substantially reduced. Similar observations have been made with respect to dentistry. Jepson (1986) reports that when the dentist–patient relationship is one of co-participation, in which comprehensive discussion of treatment options and their probable outcomes are used to help patients make informed decisions about their dental health care, high levels of compliance are achieved.

Satisfaction with health care

Patients have a number of goals when they seek dental care. These include the diagnosis and treatment of any oral problems, the relief of fear and anxiety which result from those problems, and the relief of anxiety about the procedures involved in the provision of treatment. Patients judge dentists on their personal qualities rather than their technical competence and are more satisfied with those dentists who are successful at relieving anxiety. This ability depends upon the quality of the interaction between dentist and patient. Corah (1984) and Gale *et al.* (1984) have shown that limited verbal interaction between dentist and patient leads to less anxiety reduction, less positive attitudes towards the dentist, and lower levels of satisfaction with dental care. In turn, both satisfaction and anxiety are important factors influencing whether patients present for regular dental care. In this respect, a willingness to listen, to explain, and to deal with the patient's concerns are taken as an indication of a general interest in patients and their welfare, and are qualities most appreciated by patients.

The social dimensions of healing

Improving the communication between practitioner and patient has another important effect; it improves patients' physiological and psychological responses to therapy and leads to more favourable therapeutic outcomes. The 'biosocial bridges', linking the social and psychological processes involved in the doctor–patient relationship and the physiological processes of recovery from illness, have become the subject of systematic research effort.

One of the earliest studies which demonstrated this link was undertaken by Egbert *et al.* (1964), who showed quite clearly the beneficial effects of improved pre-operative communication with patients. Ninety-seven patients undergoing abdominal surgery were randomly assigned to experimental and control groups. The patients in the control group were subject to the hospital's usual pre-operative procedures, whereas those in the experimental group were visited by the anaesthetist who discussed at length the post-operative pain they should expect. These patients were informed about the location, severity and duration of the pain and reassured that such pain was normal following their type of surgery. Post-operative monitoring of both groups of patients revealed that those in the experimental group experienced less pain: they received less narcotics (see Figure 8.1), were more comfortable, in better physical and emotional condition, and left hospital on average three days earlier than the controls.

The effect of improved communication on post-operative pain has been explained by the reduction of stress and anxiety achieved by informing patients of what to expect. It has also been shown that reducing the general anxieties created by going into hospital can have equally beneficial pre- and post-operative effects. Pre-operative anxiety has an influence on the patient's physiological state, so that highly anxious patients are more difficult to anaesthetize. Managing such anxiety is necessary to maximize the patient's physiological condition prior to surgery and to reduce the dose of anaesthetic required. The results of a number of small scale studies have shown that care by a nurse specially trained in communication reduces both the stress experienced by the patient and the somatic complications which follow surgery. In a more substantial study by Skipper and Leonard (1968), eighty children having tonsillectomies were randomly assigned to experimental and control groups. The experimental group was admitted by a nurse whose specific job was to provide the mother with information and support at the time of admission, and at several stages during the child's stay in hospital. The control group were subject to the hospital's usual procedures. The results indicated that both mothers and children in the experimental group experienced less stress, which led to an improvement in the post-operative physiological state of the child. There were significant differences between

Figure 8.1 Post-operative treatment with narcotics: means for each day

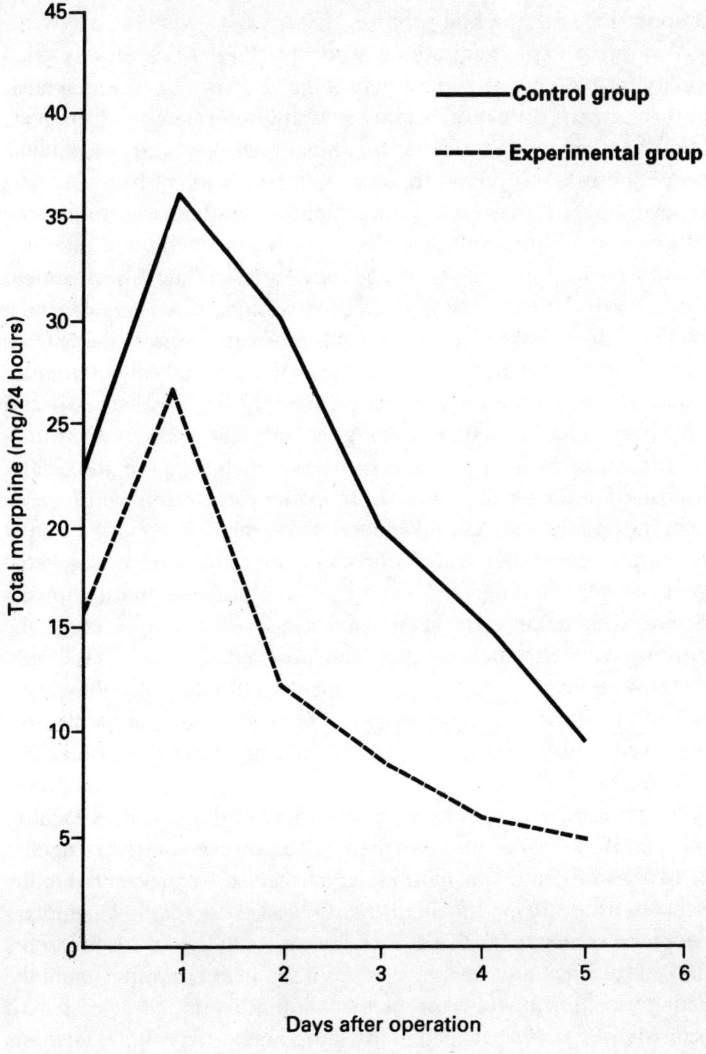

Source: Egbert *et al*. 1964

the experimental and control groups on a number of physiological measures such as blood pressure, heart rate, vomiting, voiding, and fluid consumption, indicating a more satisfactory recovery among the experimental group.

A more recent longitudinal study by Fitzpatrick *et al.* (1983) looked at patients attending neurological clinics for the diagnosis and treatment of severe headache. Using interviews with patients before and after the consultation and at follow-up one year later, a reduction in the severity, frequency and duration of headache was reported by just over half of the patients seen. This was not related to any specific therapy provided as a result of the consultation: those who were prescribed drugs showed no greater improvement than those who were not given a prescription. The variable which distinguished those who showed symptomatic improvement from those who did not was satisfaction with the original consultation in general and communication in particular. Both satisfaction and the subsequent reduction in symptom severity were related to the extent to which the neurologists' actions, including the advice and information they gave, were felt by patients to be relevant to their own individual worries and concerns. The ability to make sense of previously confusing and disturbing symptoms, and the sense of control over the illness achieved as a result of consultation with a doctor who dealt with such worries and concerns, explain the symptomatic improvement in the satisfied group. This study clearly demonstrates the social dimensions to healing and the contribution to patients' well-being made by the social as well as the diagnostic and technical aspects of the practitioner–patient relationship.

In more general terms, the results of all of these studies point to the significance of empowerment. Empowerment is a concept drawn from health promotion, and refers to a process whereby people can be helped to help themselves. This involves teaching people to recognize and deal with the causes of the health problems they encounter, and instilling in them the belief that they can take action to confront these problems. Similarly, the knowledge and information conveyed to patients empowers; it provides patients with the means to manage their illnesses more successfully and, more importantly, it gives them a sense of mastery and control over their health.

Improving communication with patients

The foregoing review should leave no doubt that improving communications is the responsibility of the practitioner. The dentist or doctor is the dominant partner in the consultation and largely determines its content and its course.

Ley (1976) has undertaken a series of experiments on comprehension and memory, and produced guidelines for improving practitioner–patient communication. These include: give advice and instructions as early as possible in the interview and stress their importance, give specific detailed information rather than general comments, use short words and sentences, and repeat essential information regarding the diagnosis and treatment.

However, failures of comprehension and memory are not the only reasons for poor communication. Consequently, Tuckett *et al.* (1985) suggest that practitioner and patient must use the consultation to work towards a shared understanding of the patient's problem. Successful shared understanding will have been achieved if the patient is able to remember the key points of what the practitioner said, interpret these points correctly and be aware of any points of conflict or difference with the practitioner and the reasons for them. This means that the practitioner's explanation of the problem and the patient's explanation of the problem must be explicitly addressed along with the ideas each has about appropriate therapy. This presupposes an awareness on the practitioner's part of patients' needs for information, and a readiness to broaden the consultation to include non-clinical as well as clinical issues. Practitioners need to be able to recognize the often subtle ways patients attempt to convey their own ideas, worries, and concerns and to create opportunities for these to be expressed. The goal of a consultation is not simply one of arriving at a diagnosis and formulating a treatment plan; patients need to be offered the means whereby they can make sense of and develop a sense of control over their illness and its course. To the extent that this is achieved, the full therapeutic benefits of the encounter will be realized.

9
The sociology and psychology of pain

Pain is a common experience in daily life. Data presented in other chapters have revealed that oral and facial pain is reported by a significant proportion of the population. Pain is also one of the symptoms most frequently encountered in dental practice and a frequent accompaniment to the clinical procedures involved in the diagnosis and treatment of oral disease. Many people avoid visiting the dentist because of a fear of pain (Liddell and May 1984). Although there have been major developments in our understanding and appreciation of pain, it remains something of a mystery. Without doubt, it is a complex phenomenon and involves neurological, physiological, and psychological components. It is one area of study where the traditional distinction between biology and psychology becomes blurred and difficult to justify.

Pain is difficult to define and even more difficult to quantify. It is essentially a private and personal experience which is only made available to others by means of verbal expression or pain-related behaviours. However, not all individuals experience pain in the same way. Social and cultural factors affect attitudes and expectations regarding pain, and these influence the way in which pain is perceived and communicated to others.

The nature of pain

A useful point of departure for a discussion of the nature of pain is to be found in the definition offered by Merskey and Spear (1967: 9). They consider pain to be 'an unpleasant experience which we primarily associate with tissue damage or describe in terms of tissue damage or both.' While somewhat ambiguous in its characterization of pain, this definition implies a biological or disease model of pain. It suggests that pain is organic in origin, and that once the cause of the noxious stimulus is identified, the pain can be removed by surgical or other means. Clinical experience indicates that this view of pain has a lot to recommend it. Pain is caused by tissue damage and clinical intervention is often, if not always, successful in relieving it.

However, other observations and the results of experimental studies suggest that there is more to pain than is implied by the disease model. There is not, for example, a direct relationship between the amount of tissue damage and the intensity of pain experienced. Pain does not always follow from tissue damage nor does pain always have a verifiable organic cause. This means that an understanding of the physiological aspects of pain is insufficient to understand pain or people in pain.

Some of the earliest and most vivid observations contributing to what has been called 'the puzzle of pain' were reported by Beecher (1956). His experience as a field anaesthetist during World War II revealed that many soldiers who had been severely wounded reported only slight pain or seemed to feel no pain at all. This was in complete contrast to the civilian patients treated by Beecher during his practice prior to the war, who reported severe pain from post-operative wounds of similar severity. Only 25 per cent of soldiers requested pain relief compared to 90 per cent of the civilians. Beecher initially thought that this might be due to a certain stoicism on the part of the soldiers and a general reluctance to make their pain known. He found, however, that they were quite willing to compain about the relatively minor discomfort involved in an injection, and subsequently rejected the explanation that the differences observed were due to differences in behavioural responses to pain. Other clinical observations are equally puzzling. For example, there is no direct relationship between the amount of pain women report during childbirth and obstetric indicators of the degree of difficulty associated with the birth (Uddenberg 1979). Labour time, birth weight and head circumference are not good predictors of the amount of pain experienced. Similarly, there is no relationship between the diameter of the needle used during a dental injection and the amount of pain reported by the patient.

Beecher concluded that the magnitude of an injury was not the key factor in terms of the level of pain experienced. Rather, it was the situation in which the pain occurred which influenced pain perception. A soldier was likely to view even a severe injury with relief since it led to his removal from the field of battle and the greater threat of death. For a civilian, a surgical operation was more likely to be viewed as a threatening and anxiety-provoking event and accompanied by fears of its implications for the future. This explanation is consistent with anthropological observations in which severe injuries inflicted as part of religious ceremonies appear to cause little pain. Similarly, injuries sustained as an essential part of initiation or manhood rites do not seem to cause the expected degree of pain and athletes often continue to play the game seemingly unaware of broken bones or other injuries.

Even more damaging to the disease model of pain is the phenomenon known as phantom limb pain. Some patients who have had a limb removed continue to experience pain in that limb even though it is no longer there. Because it is persistent and does not respond well to conventional treatment methods, this kind of pain can be very distressing for both clinician and patient. It is also the case that pain can be experienced by patients with transection of the spinal cord in parts of the body without a viable nerve supply.

These observations not only challenge the disease model of pain, they reveal severe deficiencies in the organic approach to the treatment of pain. This organic approach leads to an over-emphasis on the source of pain rather than the pain itself. As a result, the clinician may dismiss patients who complain of pain in the absence of any demonstrable organic cause, or patients whose complaints appear to be inconsistent with the degree of injury or tissue damage involved. A broader approach, based on a more holistic view of pain, indicates that the objective should be the treatment of the patient's *experience* of pain as well as of the organic source of that experience.

The gate theory of pain

In an attempt to explain the above and other observations, Melzack and Wall (1965) developed the gate theory of pain. This theory introduced social and psychological factors into the pain experience and described the neurophysiological processes by means of which these factors exert their influence. Although the theory has not been universally accepted, it provides a useful framework for understanding pain and suggests alternative mechanisms for the control of pain.

According to Melzack and Wall, pain is multifaceted and involves a sensory–discriminative component, an affective–motivational component and a cognitive–evaluative component. The first consists of sensory information regarding the location and magnitude of an injury or assault on the body, the second consists of the perceived meaning of and emotional response to these sensations, and the third involves past experience and culturally determined expectations. These components interact to determine the nature of the pain episode and, ultimately, behavioural responses to pain. As Melzack states:

> Pain is a perceptual experience whose quality and intensity is influenced by the past history of the individual, the meaning he gives to the pain-producing situation, and by his state of mind at the moment. Pain becomes a function of the whole individual, including his present thoughts and fears, as well as his hopes for the future. (Melzack 1973: 22)

Melzack and Wall described the neurophysiological basis of the pain experience in the following way. Sensory nerve fibres transmit nerve impulses from all parts of the body to the spinal cord. Two types of fibres are involved in this process: large-diameter fibres which conduct non-painful tactile stimuli and small fibres which conduct impulses from receptors which are activated by high-intensity stimuli. The nerve impulses transmitted by these fibres enter the dorsal horns of the spinal cord and activate transmission cells located in those horns. In turn, these cells relay information up the spinal cord to the brain by means of ascending nerve pathways. When the volume of impulses sent out by the transmission cells reaches a certain level, the stimuli at the peripheral sites are experienced as pain. The strength of the incoming impulses from peripheral sites is dependent upon the number of sensory nerve fibres involved and the rate of impulse transmission. In turn these influence the output of the dorsal horn transmission cells. If this were the only mechanism involved then there would be a more direct relationship between the magnitude of tissue damage, the strength of the incoming stimuli, and the level of pain experienced. However, Melzack and Wall suggest that this process is influenced by a gate mechanism which determines the level of activity of the dorsal horn transmission cells.

This gate control mechanism may be influenced by incoming impulses from peripheral sites and descending impulses from the brain. Nerve impulses transmitted along large-diameter nerve fibres inhibit the activity of the dorsal horn cells while impulses from small fibres stimulate transmission cell activity and open the gate. Transmission cell output and pain sensations are dependent upon the ratio of large to small fibre transmission. Mild peripheral stimulation increases large fibre transmission and dampens the transmission cell response. Where these fibres are damaged by disease or injury small fibre impulses dominate and open the gate to pain transmission. Melzack and Wall use this model to account for phantom limb pain. They believe that the loss of a limb removes both large and small fibres and, in the absence of inhibition, the dorsal horn gate remains permanently open.

The gate mechanism also responds to impulses from the brain. Attention, memory, and emotions are selectively triggered by incoming pain impulses emanating from the spinal cord. Central systems activated by these processes produce downwardly conducted impulses which influence the gate by diminishing or amplifying transmission cell activity. This is the mechanism by means of which psychological processes influence the quality and intensity of the pain. For example, it is suggested that fear and anxiety excite the dorsal horn cells receiving peripheral messages and enhance the pain experience.

According to the gate theory, the relationship between the magnitude of tissue damage and pain is mediated by central nervous system activity. Minor tissue damage may result in what appears to be a disproportionate level of pain if the gate is opened as a result of psychological processes. Variation in individual and situational factors will mean that what is painful to one person will not be to another. Equally, a given stimulus may produce more pain in one context than in another. Paradoxically, this should mean that the results of experimental studies on pain undertaken in the laboratory may not be applicable to clinical or real life situations. This is because the laboratory and real life are different in a number of ways, all of which will have a bearing on the respective pain experiences of participants and patients. For example, subjects in pain experiments are usually volunteers, they know that the pain they experience will be short-lived, and they know that they can ask for the pain to be terminated should it rise to intolerable levels. These factors will significantly influence attitudes to pain and, in turn, pain perception. Moreover, pain is usually induced by stimuli which do not appear in everyday life, so that the effect of prior experience and emotional reactions to the stimulus itself will be considerably reduced. Consequently, people exposed to a stimulus in a laboratory situation should experience less pain than people exposed to the same stimulus but in a clinical situation. This is precisely what happens. Dworkin and Chen (1982) administered a series of electric shocks to the incisors of a group of volunteers. Half were given the shocks in a laboratory setting, while half were given shocks in a clinical setting by a dentist. The latter began to report pain at lower levels of electric shock and reached their pain threshold (the maximum pain that could be endured) earlier.

Another interesting finding is that morphine is far more effective in relieving natural pain than experimental pain. This is probably due to the anxiety-reducing properties of morphine and the different levels of anxiety experienced by patients and subjects in experiments. The latter are less likely than the former to be anxious about the pain they experience.

Social and psychological factors and the pain experience

In any discussion of the social and psychological factors which influence the experience of pain, it is important to draw a distinction between what a person feels and what a person does, between the pain *sensation* and pain *behaviour* (Helman 1984). Both may be influenced by a range of social and psychological factors. For example, cultural differences in the significance attached to pain may modify the severity of pain experienced and the behavioural response to pain.

Evidence would suggest that pain is, in part, a learned response. This learning takes a number of forms. There are, for example, cultural differences in definitions of what constitutes pain, and in the expectation and acceptance of pain as a normal facet of life. Zborowski (1952) has compared the perception of labour pain in Poland and the US. In the former, such pain is both expected and accepted and does not give rise to requests for analgesics. In the US, it is more likely to be viewed as an unnecessary and unwelcome accompaniment to childbirth and subject to chemotherapeutic control. Such definitions are learned within the family, with attitudes about pain and pain responses being transmitted from parents to children. Even within a given culture, individual differences may occur as a result of a family's own mode of coping with pain.

There is some experimental evidence to suggest that the response of others affects both sensitivity to pain and the propensity to report pain. For example, dogs raised in isolation do not respond 'normally' to supposedly painful stimuli. Unlike dogs raised in groups, they show no apparent distress and do not learn to avoid such stimuli even after many encounters. In an experiment conducted by Craig and Prkachin (1978), the pain tolerance of a group of volunteers was tested by subjecting them to electric shocks and obtaining verbal ratings of the level of pain experienced using a numerical scale. Unknown to these subjects one individual had been instructed to give artificially low pain ratings. This group reported less pain than another group who had not been thus exposed, and were also less able to distinguish between shocks of different intensity. From this Craig and Prkachin concluded that the responses of others influence pain sensations as well as pain behaviour.

Another type of learning is to be found in previous experience. An event that proved to be painful in the past will give rise to the expectation that it will be painful when encountered in the future and may, therefore, *be* more painful. Burstein and Burstein (1979) studied the pain produced by dental injections and found that past experience, expectations, and the pain reported following such an injection were highly associated.

Situational influences and the pain experience

The link between the past and the present in terms of pain is most likely to be found in anxiety. The expectation of pain creates anxiety about pain and leads to the sensation of pain following an encounter with the noxious stimulus in question. Anxiety is one of the most important components of the pain experience. According to Dworkin *et al.* (1978) the relationship between anxiety and pain is simple and direct: the more anxious an individual then the greater his or her propensity to perceive pain. So powerful is the influence of anxiety that it frequently overrides any variations in response due to cultural factors. Even in the laboratory context anxiety plays a prominent role, with anxious subjects more likely to characterize various stimuli as painful than those who are not anxious. Since encounters with dentists and the treatments which constitute dental care often provoke anxiety, the clinical setting itself may serve to heighten the patient's awareness of pain.

In Chapter 8 mention was made of the links between anxiety, information, and pain. The relationship is not unidirectional but reciprocal. This loop effect can be broken only if special procedures are used to reduce or eliminate any or all of these. In a treatment setting a number of factors will determine the amount of anxiety experienced by the patient. These are:

1 the extent to which the patient understands what is going to happen;

2 the extent to which the patient can predict the course of any discomfort or other sensations experienced;

3 the extent to which the patient accepts the treatment;

4 the meanings attached to any sensations experienced; and

5 the degree to which the patient feels in control of what is happening.

Clearly, the solution to the problem of anxiety rests in the dentist–patient relationship. An awareness of the patient's psychological needs and a willingness to provide for those needs constitute the basis for controlling pain perception and behaviours during dental treatment.

Cultural differences in pain behaviour

Cultural factors influence not only the perception of pain but also the response to pain. They will have an impact on an individual's willingness to report pain, the manner in which pain is communicated to others, and requests for action with respect to pain. Differences in pain behaviours will be observed with respect to modes of verbal expression, changes in demeanour and activity, and expectations for help and support. By and large, these differences are the product of cultural variations in the meaning and significance attached to pain and attitudes to the sharing of suffering.

Pain is essentially private and only becomes public when displayed verbally or non-verbally. In some cultures, particularly those which value stoicism and the suppression of feelings and emotion, pain may remain private. Here the absence of pain behaviours cannot be taken to mean the absence of pain. Within cultures there may be differences in terms of who is expected to display pain and who is not. This is more likely to apply to men than to women, and considerable social status may be acquired by those who are able to remain silent in the face of pain. These cultural differences in pain expression may lead to misunderstandings in the practitioner–patient relationship and an inappropriate clinical response. The pain of the stoic may not be revealed and addressed, while the pain of those who respond with an emotional display may be dismissed or given a psychiatric diagnosis. In cultures where the display of emotional as opposed to physical distress is not encouraged, psychiatric conditions such as depression or acute anxiety may present as pain, which is a more socially acceptable complaint. In other cases, pain provides an entry to the practitioner–patient relationship and may be the first step in the process of mobilizing help. However, the likelihood of help being given depends upon the fit between the symptoms, the way they are expressed by the sufferer, and the social values of the group to which the individual belongs (Zola 1966). When dealing with patients in pain, the attitudes and values of the clinician must be put aside and the pain behaviour viewed in terms of its cultural context. If seen through an inappropriate frame of reference, it is unlikely that the patient's problem will be fully understood and the right kind of therapy or help offered.

The early study by Zborowksi (1952) remains the most detailed and illuminating account of the relationship between culture and pain. He observed marked differences in pain responses between three hospitalized groups: Italian Americans, Jewish Americans, and Protestant 'Old Americans'. Patients of Italian and Jewish extraction tended to be very emotional in the expression of their pain, while the 'Old Americans' tended to adopt a more detached approach and, when asked about their pain, described its character, location, and timing rather than the degree of distress it caused.

The similar emotional displays of the Italian and Jewish Americans were in fact based on different cultural attitudes to pain. The Italians were concerned with the immediate pain experience itself, but once their pain was relieved they reverted to normal patterns of behaviour. The Jewish Americans were mainly concerned with the meaning and significance of the pain for their own future welfare and that of their families. Even after the pain had been relieved they remained worried and concerned about its underlying cause. Some continued to complain about the pain in order to ensure that the origins of the pain received sufficient attention as well. In this respect the function of the pain behaviour was quite different and directed towards different ends. Zola (1966) also noted differences between the presentation of symptoms by Italian and Irish Americans. The supposedly exaggerated responses of the former seemed to result in a greater frequency of psychiatric diagnoses in those cases where no organic cause was found to account for the symptoms.

Strategies for pain control

A wide range of strategies for pain control are available to the dental practitioner and these range from the mundane, to the exotic, to the invasive. Clinical approaches include the use of drugs or surgery, while psychological approaches include relatively simple cognitive techniques, hypnosis, and, arguably, acupuncture. The techniques selected will vary according to the individual patient, the practitioner's skills and resources, and the type of pain that needs to be relieved, whether acute or chronic, pathogenic or iatrogenic. In many cases, the judicious use of one or more techniques is most effective. For example, there is some evidence to suggest that pain relief using chemical agents works better if used in conjunction with techniques designed to reduce anxiety (Dworkin *et al.* 1978). The most common type of pain encountered in general dental practice is that associated with operative procedures such as injections, fillings, and extractions. Here psychological techniques are the most appropriate unless the patient's anxiety is so pronounced that some form of sedation must be considered. Effective interpersonal relations are a powerful tool which can enhance considerably the quality of care given.

The pain control techniques available to the general practitioner can be classified according to which component of the pain experience they attempt to modify (Kent 1984). Strategies aimed at the sensory-discriminative aspect of pain include surgical procedures to destroy nerve pathways, blocking of neural transmission by drugs, external stimulation, and relaxation. Surgical procedures are only used in special cases of intractable pain, while locally active preparations such as Novocaine are a routine feature of dental practice. These drugs need to be distinguished from other compounds such as morphine, which appear to affect the central systems responsible for the emotional and evaluative aspects of pain. Relaxation can reduce pain by relieving tension and dampening the activity of the sympathetic nervous system. There is some evidence to suggest that training in relaxation can increase tolerance to pain and can be useful in situations where the fear of pain prevents the individual from seeking dental care (Klepac 1975).

Techniques which address the affective-motivational and cognitive-evaluative components of pain attempt to modify the individual's perception and interpretation of the sensory input experienced. Strategies involving *distraction* aim to reduce the level of attention paid to the sensations being received and are based on the assumption that when a person's attention is directed towards a painful stimulus the pain becomes more intense. It is a common observation that people caught up in activities which require concentration are often unaware of pain. Similarly, many people in pain report that it is more severe at night when the activities of everyday life are not there to distract them. Early efforts at distraction involved the use of 'audio-analgesia'; that is, using music or 'white noise' to divert the patient's attention away from pain. Although some experimental studies have produced impressive results, it is now believed that this approach needs to be used in combination with suggestion in order to provide a worthwhile level of pain relief for most patients. Other examples of distraction would be asking the patient to perform some mental task while under treatment or asking them to use *selective attention*. The latter involves focusing on some positive aspect of the situation giving rise to pain in order to bring about a reinterpretation of the meaning of that situation. In the case of dental patients, this might be benefits such as better oral health, improved aesthetics, or the reduction of the likelihood of future pain. Experimental and clinical studies have shown positive results with this technique.

A strategy that can help to modify the emotional connotations of a painful stimulus is the use of neutral rather than highly charged words. If the language used in describing procedures to patients is not carefully selected then the expectation of pain may be generated and sensations associated with the procedure experienced as pain. Experimental studies have shown that when volunteers are subjected to unpleasant stimuli and told that they will be painful, they score more highly on both self-report and physiological measures of pain than participants with whom the word 'pain' has not been used. In the clinical situation, patients must be told about the kind of sensations they can expect to experience. A failure to inform or attempts to mislead the patient will have negative consequences for the patient–practitioner relationship and diminish the trust on which the relationship must be based. However, it does not take much imagination to offer the patient descriptions which, while accurate, do not create the kind of anxieties or expectations which exacerbate pain.

A final strategy which is easy to use within the dental surgery involves transferring a degree of control over what is taking place to the patient. Laboratory studies have shown that the tolerance of the pain of electric shocks increases when the participants are given control over the timing and intensity of those shocks. Clinical studies by Wardle (1982a) and Thrash *et al.* (1982) have shown that this approach is effective in reducing the discomfort patients experience during injections or routine dental care. The control given to these patients took the form of a simple signal, such as the raising of an arm, which was used to instruct the dentist to stop whatever he or she was doing. This technique seems to reduce patients' fears that they will experience severe and inescapable pain.

The placebo effect

The placebo effect is a major component of all therapies and not just pain control techniques. It can be defined as 'any effect attributable to a pill, potion or procedure but not its pharmacodynamic or specific properties' (Wolf 1959: 698). Simply put, it is the positive effects of drugs or procedures which stem from the patient's belief in their efficacy. These positive effects are almost invariably observed when the drug or procedure is an inert substance or apparent rather than real.

According to Claridge (1970), the *total drug effect* depends upon a number of factors other than its pharmacological characteristics. These include the physical attributes of the drug, the characteristics of the patient receiving the drug, the personality or authority of the person prescribing the drug, and the setting in which the drug is administered. The placebo effect can be understood as the total drug effect minus any active properties of the drug itself. Placebos have been reported to provide relief from a wide range of physical and psychological disorders; they can also produce side effects and dependency.

The exact mechanism by which placebos work is not fully understood, although the process is likely to be a psychophysiological one. Since the analgesic properties of placebos disappear when patients are given naloxone, it has been hypothesized that their effects are produced by the secretion of endorphins or endogenous opiates. However, since it appears that placebos are culture-bound, that is, they are dependent upon the setting in which they are given, then a major component of their effect must be psychological. Anthropologists would see their effects as being rooted in systems of belief and ritual, so that placebos which work in one cultural or social group may not work in another.

The nature and extent of the placebo effect, whether associated with an active preparation or an inert substance, is largely dependent upon the practitioner–patient relationship. Rapport, mutual confidence, and shared expectations and understandings are necessary for the placebo effect to be observed. The patient's knowledge of and attitudes towards drugs and what they have been told about the preparation they are taking can diminish or enhance the placebo effect. The sense of anxiety, vulnerability, and dependency which almost invariably accompanies pain or illness also renders the individual more prone to the placebo effect. The characteristics of the practitioner are also crucial. The authority of the prescriber, the confidence he or she inspires, and his or her ability to manipulate the patient's beliefs or expectations will determine the degree of relief obtained. In this regard, healing involves important symbolic and ritual elements which, combined with the direct impact of drugs or other procedures, are necessary to the patient's physical and psychological well-being (Helman 1984).

10

Fear and anxiety

Fear and anxiety are common responses to anticipated or actual dental treatment. This may range from extreme anxiety long before treatment is happening to slight feelings of unease during procedures such as an injection or the preparation of a cavity. Estimates of the proportion of the adult population who are anxious about dental care range from 5 to 30 per cent. In spite of these differences in estimates of the prevalence of dental anxiety, there is general agreement and research evidence to show that it constitutes a major problem for the dentist and a barrier to optimal oral care.

One of the most significant consequences of fear and anxiety is avoidance of necessary dental treatment. In a national study of adults in the UK, two fifths said that they only ever went to the dentist if they were having pain or other trouble with their teeth. Of these, almost 60 per cent reported that part of the reason was their fear of the dentist and dental treatment (Todd *et al.* 1982). Essentially similar results were reported by Liddell and May (1984). They found that irregular attenders scored significantly higher on a test measuring dental anxiety than did regular attenders. Fear and anxiety are also associated with delay in seeking treatment. In a study of patients attending an emergency clinic because of pain, Segal (1986) found that 15 per cent had been in constant pain for a month or more. This may mean more extensive treatment when they do present which may, in turn, merely serve to exacerbate their fear of dentistry. Curson and Coplans (1970) found that relatively few dentally anxious patients who finally requested emergency care made and kept further appointments for the non-emergency treatment they required.

Although fear and anxiety are significant barriers to the seeking of care many patients do accept treatment in spite of their worries and concerns. A study of 750 general practice patients in Wales found that 32 per cent were slightly anxious about dental treatment and 14 per cent were very anxious. Most of these located the source of their anxiety in their previous experience of dental care (Green and Green 1985). The study suggests that fearful patients are a routine part of the dental practitioner's working day. Other studies indicate that such patients show more resentment towards dentists and are less satisfied with the care they receive. In this respect, fear and anxiety leading to infrequent or delayed dental treatment create both clinical and interpersonal problems for the dentist. Certainly, practising dentists report that such patients are a common and major source of stress (see Chapter 12).

The nature of dental fear and anxiety

Fear and anxiety are complex and, to some extent, overlapping psychological states that are difficult to define precisely. Anxiety can be defined as a vague, unpleasant feeling accompanied by a premonition that something undesirable is about to happen. This sense of unease or discomfort can have physiological and behavioural consequences. Where a distinction is drawn between anxiety and fear, the former is taken to refer to a general sense of threat, whereas the latter refers to a specific situation, object, or event. Fear is often defined as the anticipation of threat or harm elicited by an identifiable source.

One of the problems with anxiety is that it is strongly associated with the unknown. While anxious people know that they are experiencing psychological discomfort they are often unable to explain why. Their anxiety frequently seems to have no rational or objectively verifiable cause. In fact, anxiety may persist even when the individual knows that there is little or no danger involved. People who are anxious about flying know that the chances of harm are minimal, but this does little to relieve their anxiety. One of the problems people have in dealing with anxiety is that behaviours which make it possible to lessen their sense of threat are difficult to identify. Here total avoidance becomes the only way of coping with their feelings. Because the sources and consequences of fear are objectively verifiable, fear reduction is easier to achieve through rational explanation and coping behaviour (Dworkin *et al.* 1978).

The kinds of dental procedures which provoke anxiety have been studied by Gale (1972), Jackson (1978) and Wardle (1982b). As anticipated, invasive procedures such as extractions, injections, and cavity preparation were more likely to be judged to be sources of anxiety than non-invasive procedures. In their study of 419 adults, mostly women, Lindsay *et al.* (1987) found that 30 per cent were very or extremely anxious about fillings and 28 per cent were similarly anxious about oral injections. Gale (1972) divided his subjects into high and low fear groups based on their responses to questions about visiting the dentist. Both were asked to rank common dental procedures from most feared to least feared. Table 10.1 shows that virtually identical rankings were obtained from the two groups despite the differences in their expressed levels of anxiety about dental treatment. While the groups agreed about the *relative* unpleasantness of these procedures, they provoked anxiety of different magnitudes.

Table 10.1 Ranking of dental situations from the most feared to the least feared for high fear and low fear groups

Situation	Low fear	High fear
Dentist is pulling your tooth	1	2
Dentist is drilling your tooth	2	1
Dentist tells you that you have bad teeth	3	3
Dentist holds syringe in front of you	4	6
Dentist is giving you an injection	5	4
Have a probe placed in a cavity	6	5
Dentist laughs as he/she looks in your mouth	7	10
Dentist squirts air into a cavity	8	7
Sitting in dentist's waiting room	9	8
Dentist is laying out instruments	10	13
Nurse tells you it's your turn	12	9
Getting in the chair	11	11
Dentist is putting in the filling	13	14
Thinking about going to the dentist	15	12
Dentist cleans your teeth with probe	14	15

Source: Gale 1972. Adapted

Other studies suggest that even the non-invasive aspects of dental care can produce emotional reactions in some patients. Some edentulous people avoid going to the dentist because of fear, even though they are likely to be subject to a far narrower range of procedures and objectively less threatening treatments than the dentate (Todd *et al.* 1982). Nine per cent of those interviewed by Lindsay *et al.* (1987) found scaling and polishing provoked extreme anxiety. Even the anticipation of dental care is highly stressful for patients at the extreme end of the dental fear scale. These studies indicate that anxiety and fear are not totally explained by the *type* of procedures patients expect or are subjected to. The non-specific aspects of the dental situation seem to provoke anxiety in some. This view is also supported by research on children which failed to find any relationship between the number or type of dental procedures given to twelve-year-olds over a three-year period and subsequent levels of dental anxiety (Murray 1987). Consequently, the emotional response to dental care cannot be readily predicted from the actual treatments provided.

Another interesting set of results has emerged from studies which have documented age and sex differences in dental fear and anxiety. In a survey of dental care utilization undertaken in the US, 18 per cent of adults avoided dentists because of fear compared to 5 per cent of children under the age of thirteen years. When avoidance was examined by sex, different results emerged for children and adults. Boys were more likely than girls to avoid treatment because of fear, whereas women were more likely to avoid dental care than men.

In a major review of research on children and dental anxiety, Winer (1982) concluded that while the majority of younger children appeared to be cooperative in dental settings there was an increase in dental fear with age. Liddell (1985) studied a group of children at age nine and again at age twelve and found a significant increase in anxiety over the intervening period, with girls contributing more than boys to the increase. Other studies have also noted higher levels of dental anxiety in adolescent girls when compared to adolescent boys (Kleinknecht *et al.* 1973). Winer suggested that age-related changes in dental anxiety coincided with other physiological and psychological changes. For example, changes in endocrine functioning occur, along with increased cognitive sophistication and sensitivity to the interactional aspects of dental treatment, such as the dentist's personality, manner, and competence. Older children have also shown a heightened concern with bodily injury. It is also the case that older children visit the dentist more frequently, are more likely to have received extensive restorative care and are, therefore, more likely to have suffered pain or discomfort during treatment. In this case, greater anxiety may be rooted in a greater degree of experience with dentistry.

Age-related differences in the quality of the interaction with dentists may also play a role. Older children or the dentally experienced may receive less information and less support than younger children because the dentist perceives less anxiety on their part. Overt manifestations of anxiety, for example, are known to decrease with age. These interactional differences may also help explain sex differences in dental anxiety. Ackerman (1987) found that male dentists were better able to estimate the anxiety levels of their male than their female patients.

The origins of dental anxiety

Early attempts to account for the origins of dental anxiety focused on biological differences, personality differences, and unconscious psychological conflicts. Relatively little convincing evidence has emerged to support the causal role of these factors, although one study did find personality differences between anxious and non-anxious children and also found a higher prevalence of emotional and behavioural disorders in the former (Lautch 1971). More convincing explanations are to be found in previous negative or traumatic experiences and various types of learning.

Support for the role of previous negative experiences is to be found in a number of studies. Lautch (1971) compared dental phobics and non-phobics and found that all the former but less than a third of the latter could recall at least one unpleasant experience with a dentist. In a larger study of children, Shaw (1975) found that anxious children were more likely than the non-anxious to have had an extraction at their first visit to the dentist and to have found this a disturbing experience.

Kleinknecht (1978) undertook a more detailed investigation and attempted to identify those features of the dental situation which were important in the formation of attitudes towards dentistry. Using essays about childhood experiences written by students, the dentist's behaviour and personality, and pain on receiving injections, were all cited by dentally anxious participants, with uncaring, cold, and impersonal behaviour on the part of the dentist being the most frequently recorded. The study also suggested that pain during childhood dental visits did not give rise to long-term fear and anxiety when treatment was provided by a dentist who was perceived as caring and friendly.

However, not all of those who score highly on dental anxiety scales can report a negative previous experience, which suggests that other factors also play a part. Learning, which has a tremendous influence on human behaviour throughout the life span, is one such factor. The family is the most important source of learning during childhood, but as a child grows peer groups begin to have more impact on attitudes, beliefs and behaviour. A number of studies have offered convincing evidence that negative attitudes and anxiety about dental care can be transmitted to a child by others. Forgione and Clarke (1974) found that relatives of dentally anxious patients had more negative attitudes to dentistry and were more likely to report traumatic dental experiences than the relatives of those who showed little or no anxiety. There also seems to be a very strong association between anxiety on the part of the mother and dental anxiety in the child. Shaw (1975) found that mothers of anxious children were themselves more likely to be dentally anxious, and Johnson and Baldwin (1968) found that children with mothers who related high on a measure of anxiety were significantly more likely to exhibit negative behaviours during dental treatment. In fact, 86 per cent of the children of anxious mothers were negatively rated on the basis of their behaviour compared to 19 per cent of children whose mothers were not anxious. However, subsequent studies indicate that this relationship may hold for the first dental visit only; negative behaviour became less frequent following greater experience with dental care.

Other types of learning may also play a role in the development of dental anxiety. Kent (1984) has suggested that the type of learning called 'classical conditioning' can be important with respect to fear and anxiety. Pavlov-type experiments have shown that the frequent association of an object and a negative event can lead to arousal and fear when the object alone is subsequently encountered. This fear may also be generalized to other objects of a similar nature. Repeated physically or emotionally traumatic experiences during dental care could produce a more or less permanent negative reaction to dental treatment. It would seem that negative experiences of medical care or hospitalization can be generalized to dentistry and result in dental anxiety.

There is also research evidence to suggest that dental anxiety may be heightened or even created within the dental situation by a failure to recognize the psychological needs of patients. Even those who are non-anxious may become anxious at times. This may happen during the first visit to a new dentist or during a procedure that the patient has not experienced before. This situational anxiety is largely the product of uncertainty. Experiments suggest that the threat of pain is more anxiety-provoking than the certainty of pain and pain itself. Consequently, the failure to address or help the patient cope with uncertainty can make dental treatment more of a negative experience for *all* patients.

The recognition and assessment of dental anxiety

Given the significance of anxiety for the practice of dentistry it is crucial that the practitioner is able to detect and assess the severity of anxiety among patients. A number of methods of measuring anxiety have been developed for research purposes, some of which can be easily applied in the dental surgery.

Some formal method of assessment is often necessary since it is not always the case that the patient's anxiety is readily apparent. As with other types of phobia, the dentally anxious may not readily admit to their problem for fear of embarrassment or ridicule.

Self-report measures

The simplest way of measuring anxiety is by means of self-report scales. This may consist of asking the patient nothing more than whether they are anxious or, if a more detailed or precise measure is required, having the patient complete an anxiety questionnaire. A number of questionnaires have been designed which measure anxiety in general and dental anxiety in particular. Some of the instruments which address general anxiety draw a distinction between *trait* anxiety and *state* anxiety. The former represents a general personality characteristic, while the latter is a more transient state induced by a certain event or situation. This type of anxiety is fluid and variable. These questionnaires have been used in the assessment of dental anxiety and seem able to distinguish the anxious from the non-anxious patient and to identify changes in anxiety levels before and after dental treatment.

The other questionnaires were specifically designed to measure dental anxiety. One of the best known is the Dental Anxiety Scale (Corah 1969). This consists of four questions, for each of which the patient is asked to pick one of five alternative answers. Each answer is given a score from 1 to 5 and the overall anxiety score

Table 10.2 The Dental Anxiety Scale

1 If you had to go to the dentist tomorrow how would you feel about it?
- a I would look forward to it as an enjoyable experience
- b I wouldn't care one way or another
- c I would be a little uneasy about it
- d I would be afraid that it would be unpleasant and painful
- e I would be very frightened of what the dentist would do

2 When you are waiting in the dentist's office for your turn in the chair, how do you feel?

3 When you are in the dentist's chair waiting while he/she gets the drill ready to begin working on your teeth, how do you feel?

4 You are in the dentist's chair to have your teeth cleaned. While you are waiting and the dentist is getting out the instruments to scrape your teeth around your gums, how do you feel?

Questions 2 to 4 are scored on the following scale:
- a Relaxed
- b A little uneasy
- c Tense
- d Anxious
- e So anxious that I break out in a sweat or feel physically sick

Source: Corah 1969

obtained by a simple addition of these values. Scores in the low teens and above indicate patients with moderate to high levels of anxiety (see Table 10.2). More detailed scales are also available. These obtain a rating of the amount of fear associated with the individual procedures involved in dental care (Kleinknecht *et al.* 1973). Anxiety in children is generally measured using drawings, although visual analogue scales have been used (McGrath *et al.* 1985). One measure presents the child with a series of line drawings of children arranged in pairs. One of the pair is an anxious or fearful child and the other a neutral or happy child. The subject indicates which of each pair represents the way he or she feels (Venham 1979). A similar assessment procedure involves the child selecting a drawing of a face from among nine which show a range of affect from extremely negative to extremely positive (McGrath *et al.* 1985).

Physiological measures

Self-report measures are readily available, are reliable and valid, and can be used in the dental surgery without any training or specialized equipment. However, when anxiety is being measured for research purposes some prefer more objective indicators in the form of physiological changes which accompany emotional arousal. Increased heart rate, changes in galvanic skin response, and palmar sweat activity are the most common physiological parameters used as indicators of anxiety states. The heart rate, for example, has been shown to change during the course of dental treatment in response to various activities undertaken by the dentist.

Clearly, physiological measures are difficult to apply in the clinical situation since they require specialized equipment and skilled personnel to monitor it. Even when used in research they are subject to a number of limitations. First, the devices used to measure physiological parameters may cause as much anxiety as the situation being studied, and second, physiological arousal occurs with all emotional states and there is no guarantee that it is anxiety and not some other response that is being measured.

Behavioural measures

Behavioural measures of anxiety have most often been used when assessing the responses of children to dental treatment. The rationale underlying this approach seems to be that children are less likely to conceal their anxiety, so that uncooperative behaviour is a valid indicator of negative emotional arousal. Adults are generally aware of social constraints on negative behaviours and are more likely to suffer in silence. Behaviours believed to indicate anxiety and commonly included in behaviour rating scales are crying, refusal to open the mouth, a stiff or rigid posture, and the pushing away of dental instruments. Although such scales are superficially attractive, they are not easy to apply in the dental situation. In the context of research, differences in observers' recognition and recording of negative behaviours are quite common, and standardization must be employed to ensure that all are using the same criteria. Another problem is that some children show a mix of positive and negative behaviours while undergoing treatment and are difficult to classify on scales which run from 'definitely positive' to 'definitely negative'.

One problem which limits the use of this method of assessment in clinical practice is the lack of a close relationship between aversive-type behaviours and the other measures of anxiety. Behavioural measures do not correlate very highly with assessments based on subjective reports. Some very anxious patients attend regularly for dental treatment and are able to control their feelings to the extent that they appear relaxed and cooperative. Observations of adult patients both before and during dental treatment suggest that differences in behaviour between anxious and non-anxious patients are confined to the waiting area. Once in the surgery there are often no differences between them (Kleinknecht and Bernstein 1978). Consequently, where researchers have compared dentists' assessments and self-reports of anxiety the correspondence has not been very good. This indicates that assessments of anxiety should not be based on behaviour, since the meaning of that behaviour may be radically different from that assumed by the observer.

Managing the anxious patient

Patients' anxieties about dental treatment are often readily controlled by drugs. These range from orally or intravenously administered compounds which induce mild to deep sedation, to those that produce relative or general anaesthesia. While a small proportion of patients may ultimately need this kind of intervention in order to be able to tolerate dental treatment, most patients can be effectively managed using simple psychological techniques. Given the general tendency to limit the use of psychotropics and anaesthetics, all of which constitute no more than the controlled poisoning of the patient, psychological strategies should be the treatments of choice.

An understanding of the causes and consequences of dental anxiety have given rise to a number of techniques to help the patient overcome dental fear. These interpersonal therapies should be made available to all patients who are anxious about aspects of the treatment situation. Those individuals who control their anxiety and do not disrupt the treatment process should be identified and offered the benefits of the strategies outlined below. While every effort should be made to avoid inflicting pain during dental treatment, it is not possible to abolish all discomfort associated with restorative, operative or even prosthetic techniques. However, unpleasant physical sensations can be rendered tolerable and patients helped to view dental care as worthwhile even if sometimes a little unpleasant. Reducing the emotional arousal associated with the various procedures involved will facilitate this goal.

Jackson (1974) has suggested a basic approach to dental care which should be used with all patients and not just the dentally anxious. It is designed to reduce the physical and psychological discomfort associated with dental treatment and thereby minimize or prevent the development of negative emotional responses. This approach is described by the following guidelines:

1 do not inflict pain if this can be avoided;

2 if pain arises, stop work and deal with it;

3 warn patients about the likelihood of pain or discomfort;

4 be accurate in assessments of the degree of pain and discomfort the patient is likely to feel;

5 introduce the patient to new procedures slowly and carefully;

6 praise desirable behaviours but do not criticize undesirable ones; and

7 maintain a quiet and relaxed working environment.

Additional rules were suggested by Jackson, and these form the basis of some of the specific anxiety-reducing interventions described below. Some can be used with all patients, while some are more appropriate for the highly anxious. Some of these methods are similar to those used in the reduction of pain. For example, cognitive approaches such as distraction, where the aim is to shift the patient's attention away from the dental procedure to a more desirable situation, and cognitive modification, where the aim is to help the patient to place a positive interpretation on the treatment experience, are described in Chapter 9.

General strategies

Reducing the patient's uncertainty about what will happen during dental treatment is one way of reducing anxiety levels. This is easily achieved by giving patients information about what will happen and why. The information given can be technical, sensory or both. The 'Tell-Show-Do' approach is an information-giving strategy frequently used with children and it consists of the following:

1 Using simple language and a matter-of-fact style, the child is told what is going to happen before each procedure.

2 The procedure is demonstrated using an inanimate object, member of staff or the dentist him or herself. The procedure can also be shown using the child as the model but without the use of dental instruments.

3 The procedure does not begin until the child understands what will be done.

Although widely used, this procedure has been evaluated in only one study and no effect was noticed with the highly anxious child. Nevertheless, it is suggested that it be used routinely since it is in no way harmful and may be helpful to the child with lower levels of anxiety (Ingersoll 1982).

There is some evidence to suggest that the nature and amount of information given to patients should be varied according to their personality characteristics and coping styles. Some patients respond to general information only and are alarmed if detailed or graphic descriptions of dental procedures are given. In others, anxiety levels are reduced and adaptation to treatment is enhanced when the amount of information is increased (Auerbach *et al.* 1976). Unfortunately, no simple and easy guidelines for use in dental practice have yet emerged from this type of work. A simple approach would be to allow patients themselves to specify what information they would like beyond general descriptions of dental procedures.

Studies of patient satisfaction have shown that patients appreciate the time and attention involved in information giving. Patients' feelings of security and trust are enhanced if this information is given in a friendly and caring manner. Emotional support and information have been shown to be more effective than information alone in promoting adaptation to medical treatment (Fassler 1980). Emotional support is important in helping people cope with all kinds of stressful situations, and an empathetic and understanding approach on the part of the dentist serves this function. Allowing patients to exercise some control over the treatment process reinforces the view that the dentist is aware of, accepts, and is willing to deal with patients' fears. In general, patients are willing to accept the discomfort that often accompanies treatment if they believe everything is being done to minimize it. It is important to note that information and support should be given *during* dental treatment as well as before. Continuous verbal encouragement of the patient while the dentist works has been identified by patients themselves as important in anxiety reduction. In this regard, anxiety should not be considered to be an emotion the patient brings to the dental surgery but a problematic aspect of the dentist–patient relationship (O'Shea *et al.* 1986).

Specific strategies

The approach described above may not be sufficient to cope with the highly anxious patient. In this case, more specific techniques must be used. The ones most commonly employed are those of relaxation, desensitization and modelling.

Relaxation therapy aims to teach the patient to control some of the physiological changes that accompany emotional arousal. The technique derives its theoretical rationale from the hypothesis that anxiety emerges out of negative interpretations which are placed on physiological changes such as a rise in heart rate or increased muscle tension. Relaxation aims to break the loop whereby awareness of physiological arousal leads to the perception of a situation as threatening and a response in the form of anxiety. One relatively simple method, which can be accomplished either by a therapist or by a tape recording of a therapist, is called progressive muscle relaxation. Here the individual is placed in a comfortable chair and asked to close his or her eyes and breathe slowly and deeply. The patient is then asked to tense and relax major muscles in turn and then to relax muscle groups throughout the whole body, beginning with the extremities and working progressively through all muscle groups. For most people this results in a general feeling of relaxation and calm. After a number of sessions, individuals are able to achieve this state independently and no longer need the guidance of a therapist. Studies of its use in dental practice have shown that it can result in significant reductions in patient anxiety. It is attractive because it requires little specialist training and does not disrupt the office treatment routine.

Biofeedback is a related method of controlling physiological arousal. Here equipment is used to monitor physiological indicators such as muscle tension or heart rate, and feedback provided to the individual in the form of an auditory or visual signal. The individual is trained to use this signal to lower their level of arousal. Using electro-myographic (EMG) and heart rate feedback, Hirschman (1980) reduced the anxiety and stress experienced by high fear patients during dental restorative work. Interestingly, anxiety reduction occurred if the signal given indicated lowered arousal when in reality physiological indicators were rising. This seems to suggest that the effect is mediated by perception and the individual's subjective awareness of physiological changes.

Miller *et al.* (1978) compared progressive relaxation training and biofeedback based on EMG activity and found both to be equally effective in reducing anxiety. The former may be more attractive to the dental practitioner interested in using such techniques since it involves little in the way of equipment.

Desensitization is a more time-consuming and costly procedure and is best undertaken by a trained psychologist. It involves training in relaxation and progressive exposure to the anxiety-provoking stimulus in question. This exposure may be imagined or real. In the former instance, a hierarchy of threat is obtained from the person undergoing therapy. This consists of a list of those aspects of a situation perceived as threatening arranged in order from least to most feared. A state of relaxation is induced and the individual asked to visualize the least feared event on the list. Any anxiety invoked is controlled by further relaxation. Gradually the individual is taken through the hierarchy until he or she is able to remain relaxed while imagining the most feared event. Such subjects are able to remain calm even when confronted by the actual situation that provoked anxiety.

Case reports have shown that this method can be effective in enabling previously highly anxious patients to undergo dental treatment. However, studies of groups have resulted in success rates of only 60 to 65 per cent, although most of the 'failures' were helped when additional techniques were used in conjunction with desensitization. The main drawback of the method is the amount of time it requires. In an early study by Gale and Ayer (1969), the subject was given nine one-hour training sessions before he was able to receive treatment.

If fear and anxiety are learned responses then it seems reasonable to suppose that individuals can learn not to fear dental treatment by observing the actions of others. This process is referred to as modelling and has been used extensively with children, although it is also recommended for use with adults. Case reports and experimental studies have revealed that anxious children who have watched cooperative children receiving dental care are less anxious and disruptive when they themselves undergo dental treatment. The effect of modelling is enhanced if the model receives praise from the dentist, if more than one model is observed, if the models are the same age as the child in question, and if the models are initially nervous but overcome their fear and allow treatment to proceed. Melamed *et al.* (1975) have shown that modelling is equally effective whether live or filmed models are used. When used with adults, success rates of 50 to 60 per cent have been reported. This rises to 80 per cent where the technique is used with other approaches such as relaxation training.

The management of the child patient

Many of the techniques described above were developed to assist the practitioner to manage child patients. The aim is to reduce the stress of dental treatment for the child and the dental staff. This is not always easy, given that dental treatment consists of a set of strange procedures undertaken in an unfamiliar and visually threatening environment by strangers. In addition, the parents of child patients may also present a problem should they respond emotionally to distress in the child. For this reason, both the child and the accompanying parent must be approached with special care. Ingersoll (1982) has described a more extensive management programme involving the prior preparation of parent and child, and additional procedures to be used during the provision of dental treatment.

Ingersoll recommends the use of the following procedures to introduce both parent and child to the dental office:

1 an initial pre-appointment letter to assist the parent to prepare the child for dental care,

2 a 'get-acquainted' period in which the child can get to know the dentist or dental assistant in a neutral setting, and

3 a modelling film.

These simple procedures ensure that the child knows what to

expect, is familiar with one or more staff, and knows the rules for behaviour in the surgery. During this time the dentist can also talk to the parent to assess the likelihood of problem behaviour during treatment.

Once in the surgery the following principles should guide the management of the child:

1 It is generally advantageous for the parent to be present during treatment unless the parent finds this too stressful. However, the dentist should establish that the parental role is one of silent observer, and he or she should not attempt to deal with the child's fear or behaviour or interfere with the dentist's attempts to do so.

2 Distraction techniques such as videotaped material are useful, especially during long appointments.

3 Although little research effort has evaluated the effects of rewards on behaviour there are grounds to believe that they are useful in obtaining the child's cooperation.

4 Using punishment to control disruptive behaviour often exacerbates that behaviour. Although it may have short-term benefits it may cause that behaviour to increase in frequency over time. Since punishment only increases the trauma of dental treatment it is not to be recommended.

In the minority of cases where a child remains disruptive or uncooperative a behaviour modification programme which goes beyond these procedures may be necessary. The dentist should recognize that once all options have been exhausted it may be necessary to terminate treatment temporarily or perhaps permanently.

11
Dental health education

During the 1970s, prevention and health promotion began to be advocated as strategies for improving the health of populations. This approach was based on the recognition that many of the diseases responsible for premature death, for example cancer, heart disease, and stroke, could not be cured but could be prevented by changes in lifestyle and behaviour. Similarly, the major oral disorders, dental decay, and periodontal disease, can also be prevented by a strategy which emphasizes a reduction in the consumption of sugar-rich foods, increasing fluoride intake and the adoption of oral hygiene practices such as flossing and brushing. Consequently, dental health education, which aims to improve dietary habits and promote preventive oral health behaviours, has become a significant component of public health programmes designed to prevent and control dental disease.

Health education can be defined as 'any combination of learning opportunities designed to facilitate voluntary adaptations of behaviour which are conducive to health' (Green 1979). This involves providing individuals or groups with educational experiences which are intended to change or enhance behaviours and improve, or at least maintain, oral health status. Despite its apparent logic and intuitive appeal, health education in general, and dental health education in particular, have been somewhat controversial and subject to debate. As a result, three distinct perspectives have emerged, each with its own view of who should be educated to do what. The 'traditional' perspective aims to change the knowledge and attitudes of individuals or groups with a view to encouraging the adoption of health-related behaviours. This approach is commonly used in schools, institutions, or dental practice and is, perhaps, the most familiar of the three. Those who advocate a 'political' perspective argue that this traditional model, with its focus on individual decision-making, has been ineffective and unproductive. They would rather see efforts directed at community decision-makers and opinion leaders in order to promote the fluoridation of water supplies or the implementation of school-based fluoride mouthrinse programmes (Frazier 1978). Those who adhere to the 'radical' perspective also advocate action to change the environment rather than individual behaviour. However, this is to be achieved through increasing the public's knowledge of health issues and the environmental causes of ill health and teaching people how to organize politically in order to challenge health-damaging conditions in the community or the workplace (Allison 1982). An example of this latter approach would be working with community or consumer groups to pressure food manufacturers to reduce the refined sugar content of convenience foods.

While these three perspectives on health education are quite different, they should be regarded as part of a multifaceted approach which has come to be called health promotion. Health promotion involves 'any combination of health education and related organizational, economic and environmental supports for behaviour conducive to health' (US Department of Health and Human Services 1981). This encompasses health education, health legislation, social marketing, communication by the mass media, and community organization in order to bring about the environmental, social, and other changes necessary for improved health.

Since current projections suggest that health education will come to form a more significant aspect of the dental practitioner's work, this chapter is largely confined to the traditional approach and the effectiveness of strategies for changing individual behaviour. This does not mean that the criticisms of this perspective have been ignored; discussion and evaluation of these criticisms are to be found in Chapter 15.

Traditional approaches to dental health education

Human behaviour is complex as it is the outcome of many interacting forces and factors. Health education has largely been concerned with identifying ways of manipulating some of these forces in order to bring about changes in behaviour conducive to health.

Most emphasis has been placed on psychological factors such as knowledge, attitudes, beliefs and emotions, and the way these may be subject to behaviour modification techniques. Some emphasis has also been placed on what can be called 'micro-social' factors, that is, the effects on behaviour of interaction between individuals and within small groups. Most dental health education programmes based on modification of one or more of these factors have been developed for use in schools, although the principles they employ can be readily applied to patients in dental practice. A major issue, however, is the extent to which these programmes are effective in producing long-term behaviour change and an improvement in oral health.

Psychological strategies in dental health education

Psychological strategies which aim to instil or improve the oral hygiene practices of individuals or groups can be differentiated according to whether they focus upon knowledge, motivation or attitudes and beliefs.

Knowledge and information

The simplest and most basic approach relies wholly upon the provision of information about the threats to oral health and the teaching of skills necessary to avoid or cope with these threats. Patients need to know about the role of plaque in periodontal disease, how to recognize plaque and how to remove it by correct brushing and flossing techniques. This approach derives its rationale from studies which have shown that both adults and children lack basic knowledge about dental diseases and methods of prevention. For example, a national study in Finland found that fewer than 50 per cent of adults knew that loose teeth were indicative of periodontal disease and 45 per cent believed that eating fibrous foods would cure gingivitis (Markula *et al*. 1977). In a study in England, only 6 per cent of children aged 14 knew the meaning of the term 'gingivitis' and in a study of the same age group in the US, only 44 per cent knew that gingivitis was caused by plaque and as few as 4 per cent knew the purpose of flossing (Blinkhorn and Verity 1979, Walsh 1985).

Evaluation of health education programmes which rely upon the transmission of information about dental disease and methods of prevention has shown that they are often successful in improving knowledge and skills but rarely successful in bringing about changes in actual oral hygiene behaviours. Where programmes have produced significant changes in oral health behaviours or improvements in indicators such as plaque or gingivitis scores, the effects have been short term and mostly disappear after the termination of the programme.

A conclusion often drawn from these studies is that repetition of health education programmes is necesary in order to secure longer-term adherence to newly acquired behaviours. The few studies that have looked at the impact of repetition have produced conflicting results, with most showing repetition to have no substantial effect. The one study which did indicate positive outcomes was conducted within the closed and controlled environment of a military academy and cannot be generalized to other populations (Tan *et al.* 1981).

The main lesson to be learned from these efforts is that knowledge is a necessary but not a sufficient factor in changing oral health practices. Clearly, the transmission of information and skills needs to be supplemented by other strategies if more permanent behaviour change is to be accomplished. These other strategies aim to enhance motivation, to promote more positive attitudes and beliefs and to harness peer group pressure as a force for change.

Motivation

One of the most common behavioural strategies for promoting behaviour change is that of reinforcement. It depends upon the simple proposition that positive or rewarding consequences immediately following a behaviour tend to strengthen an individual's commitment to that behaviour, while negative consequences decrease the probability that it will occur again. In the context of dental health education, this means offering some kind of material or social reward to individuals who demonstrate improved oral hygiene behaviours or decreased plaque scores. Programmes which use information plus positive reinforcement are generally more successful than programmes based solely on information. Studies of both children and adults have found that positive reinforcement results in greater compliance and improvements in oral hygiene, at least in the short term. For example, Iwata and Beckford (1981) studied two groups of patients enrolled in a private practice-based oral hygiene programme costing $80. One group received a basic educational programme including plaque control techniques while the other received the same programme but with the incentive of a 25 per cent reduction in their fee if their plaque scores declined substantially. At the final visit both groups had plaque scores lower than prior to the educational intervention, although the fee-reduction group showed a greater overall improvement in oral hygiene. Moreover, at a follow-up visit six months later, the fee-reduction group had maintained these improvements while the plaque scores of the other group had returned to baseline levels. Other studies have produced more pessimistic results and suggest that rewards may be useful in initiating behaviour but cease to have any long-term effect once they are withdrawn.

Despite some uncertainty regarding their long-term outcomes, positive reinforcers do appear to be useful components of a coordinated health education strategy. For the individual dental practitioner, however, they may not be an attractive proposition, given the effort and expense of providing rewards over extended periods of time. While children may well be happy with, and respond to, a token reward, however small, identifying meaningful rewards for adults is more difficult. Of course, such rewards can take the form of praise or positive comments but these should be provided as a matter of routine.

Kegeles *et al.* (1978) have suggested that self-reinforcement and self-monitoring techniques can be employed following, or instead of, tangible rewards. Self-reinforcement means that the patient rewards him or herself (or the parent rewards the child) with an enjoyable activity once certain goals regarding oral health behaviours have been achieved. Self-monitoring involves the patient in observing and recording his or her own behaviour and its outcomes in terms of lowered plaque levels as revealed by the use of disclosing tablets. Teaching patients how to monitor the outcome of their endeavours by scoring plaque levels and/or gingival inflammation provides them with a source of positive reinforcement since they have direct evidence of their accomplishments.

Attitudes and beliefs

The idea underlying strategies based on positive reinforcement is that the individual undertakes the required behaviour in order to receive the associated reward until that behaviour becomes habitual and reinforcement becomes unnecessary. In this way, positive reinforcement is a form of extrinsic motivation. Other strategies, often referred to as cognitive approaches, are based on intrinsic motivation. This is, they aim to change the individual's perception of the value of preventive oral health behaviours by manipulating attitudes and beliefs. The intrinsic value of these behaviours and their outcomes in the form of improved oral health then becomes the motivating force behind the adoption of oral self-care practices.

This approach derives its theoretical basis from the Health Belief Model (HBM). This suggests that people indulge in preventive health behaviours because they believe that: (1) they are susceptible to the disease in question, (2) the disease is serious enough to interfere with some aspects of their lives, and (3) the disease can be prevented by their own actions and that prevention involves less economic or psychological cost than the disease itself. Although this model has received a great deal of attention it does not seem to have provided a sound basis for health education programmes. A recent study using an experimental design sought to determine whether health beliefs predicted preventive dental behaviours and whether these beliefs could be changed by health education. The Health Belief Model did not prove to be a good predictor of preventive health behaviour, nor did beliefs appear to change as a result of an educational intervention (Weisenberg *et al.* 1980). In spite of the generally poor results of approaches based on the HBM, health beliefs remain a central focus of contemporary health educational efforts. The question remains, how are they to be changed?

Fear arousal

Another approach which relies on intrinsic motivation has been the use of fear arousal. This attempts to scare individuals into regular preventive oral health behaviours by stressing the awful consequences of failing to maintain high levels of oral hygiene. On the whole, the results of studies designed to assess the effect of fear appeals have been inconclusive or inconsistent. In some studies, fear arousal had no effect or only short-term effects, in others mild fear appeals were most effective, and in others strong appeals were associated with the most favourable outcomes.

Peer group pressure

One technique which combines extrinsic and intrinsic motivation makes use of peer group influences. The aim is to enhance the perceived desirability of preventive dental behaviour by providing health education to small groups of people who know each other, obtaining the cooperation of parents, family members or friends, or using children or adolescents to present health education programmes to their peers. This approach also exploits our desire to conform to the expectations of those we interact with on a daily basis and to thereby receive positive reinforcement via peer group approval. Some success has been reported in experiments using this technique, although its independent effects have often been difficult to assess, given that it frequently forms but one component of a more comprehensive strategy.

One valuable study which clearly demonstrates the relative merits of alternative approaches is illustrated in Figure 11.1. It shows the percentage of children participating in a fluoride mouthrinse programme over a period of 20 weeks. Three groups of children were used and all received the same instruction in oral disease and preventive measures. However, one group of children were offered small amounts of money if they entered into and continued with the programme, a second group participated in two discussion groups about dental disease based on the Health Belief Model, while the third group received no additional intervention. The results showed that almost half of those given a cash incentive remained in the programme for the full 20 weeks, compared with a third of the group given information only and less than a fifth of the group participating in the discussion group.

The combined results of studies testing approaches to health education based on extrinsic and intrinsic motivation do not seem to offer grounds for optimism concerning the possibility of achieving sustained behaviour change either in schoolchildren or in dental practice patients. Behaviour change is achieved in only a minority of subjects offered a health education programme or is not sustained over time. However, these studies do tend to suggest that (1) some methods are more effective than others, (2) some methods work at least for some people some of the time, (3) interventions using a combined strategy produce the best results, and (4) interventions which are personalized seem to be more effective. These observations are integral to the patient-centred approaches

Figure 11.1 *Percentages of children in each group who complied with each stage of the mouthrinse programme*

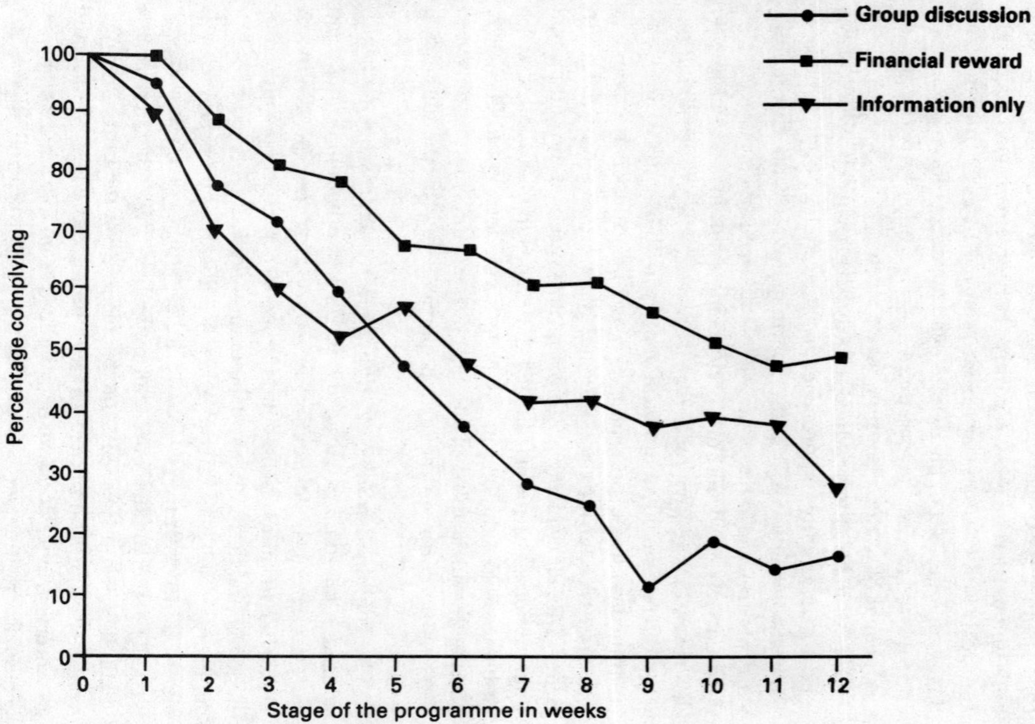

Source: Kegeles *et al.* 1978

to health education which are now advocated for use in dental practice.

At the time of writing, more sophisticated psychological theories are being used in understanding preventive oral health behaviours. An approach combining concepts from Fishbein's theory of reasoned action and Bandura's social learning theory has been shown to be more successful than other approaches in predicting positive oral health practices. This model consists of a comprehensive set of variables which address what people think and believe about behaviours. While the model has important implications for approaches to oral health behaviour change, practical strategies based on the model have yet to be developed and tested (Tedesco *et al.* 1988).

Patient-centred approaches to dental health education

Although most efforts to develop favourable oral hygiene practices among school populations or general practice patients have not produced long-term behaviour change, this does not mean that the psychological techniques outlined above should be abandoned. Rather, they should be used within a more patient-oriented strategy. This kind of approach recognizes that human behaviour is complex and not easily changed by the overly simple application of behaviour modification principles. Moreover, it recognizes that the education of patients can only proceed if the educator has a detailed understanding of the patient's perspective, and the educator and patient agree on the nature of the problem to be solved and methods to solve it. Many dentists attempt to improve the plaque control procedures of their patients before they have learned enough about the needs and goals of the patient to enable them to personalize the message (Weinstein 1982).

A study which demonstrates the benefits of a more patient-centred approach has been reported by Schou (1985). Schou designed a dental health education programme based on the following principles. Teaching was carried out in pre-existing peer groups of 5 to 7 persons in order to create a familiar and relaxed atmosphere. The teacher did not prepare a complete teaching plan but organized the content of each session in discussion with the participants. This allowed the participants to specify their own needs and goals, and ensured that they were addressed by the programme. Traditional dentist–patient roles were changed; the teacher-dentist avoided the expert role and victim-blaming behaviour, and encouraged participants to exchange their own experiences. Finally, the health education sessions were repeated at monthly intervals for five months. Measures of plaque, gingivitis, dental knowledge, and dental attitudes were taken from an experimental group subject to the programme and from a control group prior to the start of the programme and at intervals for three-and-a-half years after its termination.

The results indicated that the plaque index scores of the experimental group were significantly reduced three-and-a-half years after the completion of the programme and were significantly lower than the scores of the control group. Similarly, scores on the gingivitis index in the experimental group were significantly lower at the long-term follow-up than at baseline, while virtually no change was seen in the control group. When dental knowledge was measured six months after the completion of the health education sessions, the experimental group scored significantly higher than the controls.

Counselling techniques in general practice

When the patient-centred approach is used in general practice it is often referred to as counselling (Chiodo *et al.* 1986). Counselling draws on both behavioural and humanistic psychology and lays great emphasis on the patient–practitioner relationship, differences between patients, and the awareness, needs, and desires of patients. Weinstein and colleagues (Weinstein *et al.* 1983, 1985) have largely been responsible for the development of counselling techniques within dentistry. According to Weinstein (1982), dental health education is most successful when behaviour modification techniques are used in the context of a caring professional relationship by a dentist (or therapist) with an interest and skills in communication.

The model of behaviour change which provides the basis for the counselling approach is represented below.

Unawareness → awareness → self-interest → attitude → belief → commitment → action

Source: Blinkhorn (1981)

Perhaps the key component of this model is commitment. The

conventional approaches to health education described at the beginning of this chapter fail to take into account the extent to which people are often committed to behaviours which are damaging to health. For example, recent reports from New York indicate that many IV drug users continue to share syringes and needles in spite of possessing sterile needles provided as part of the city's efforts to prevent the spread of AIDS. The reason for this is that this sharing provides psychological benefits to the drug user which, in their own way, are as significant as the effects of the drug itself. On a more mundane level, individuals may be committed to various foods because of their psychological or social significance. The use of alcohol by adults and the sharing of sweets and candies by children, for example, offer social and psychological benefits over and above the physical pleasures associated with their consumption. This is why such behaviours can be difficult to change. On the other hand dentists are more likely to be involved in instilling desirable behaviours in their patients than in trying to extinguish undesirable ones. Nevertheless, the adoption of optimal oral hygiene practices, which are both time-consuming and tedious, requires a similar level of commitment. Assisting patients to develop the commitment to optimal oral hygiene practices is one of the main aims of counselling and is itself a time-consuming process. Counselling has been found to work in other medical settings and preliminary trials of the method suggest that it is effective in dentistry.

The counselling approach to health education consists of four distinct phases: the exploration phase, the understanding phase, the action phase and the habituation phase. Most health education efforts fail because the dentist or teacher moves directly into the action phase and neglects the first two steps in the process. The stages of the counselling process and their constituent activities are summarized in Table 11.1.

1 The exploration phase

This stage is designed to get patients to think in new ways about their oral health problems. In this phase the dentist should help the patient to recognize that a problem exists and to believe that the problem can be remedied by their own endeavours. The dentist should also establish a desire on the part of the patient to work on the problem. Health education will be ineffective if the individual does not feel that the problem is his or her own.

Table 11.1 Stages in the counselling process

1 The exploration phase

- a Establish patients' levels of knowledge, beliefs, and perceived needs
- b Establish 'ownership' of the problem

2 The understanding phase

- a Identify the nature of the problem
- b Remedy skill deficiency
- c Collect baseline data on oral hygiene performance

3 The action phase

- a Establish immediate and long-term goals
- b Implement one or more appropriate motivational strategies
- c Monitor and modify the intervention

4 The habituation phase

- a Withdraw programme in stages
- b Provide periodic review and booster sessions

Helping patients to think in new ways is not achieved by the provision of technical information concerning oral disease but through a discussion and exploration of the patient's beliefs regarding oral disease and its causes. In order to elicit these beliefs successfully, the dentist must be able to create an interpersonal environment which is non-threatening and within which the patient feels able to present his or her point of view without the fear of condemnation or criticism. The dentist needs to recognize that the patient's beliefs may not be scientifically valid but are acceptable and valid within his or her common sense ways of thinking. Accordingly, the dentist must demonstrate a respect for both the patient and his or her views. These views should not be directly challenged, nor should negative judgements be made about particular beliefs or ways of behaving. The outcome of this empathetic and receptive approach on the part of the dentist should be a caring relationship which eliminates defensiveness and maximizes the patient's receptivity to new ideas. It also enables the dentist to learn enough about a patient to personalize the subsequent stages of the process.

2 *The understanding phase*

When the patient accepts that there is a problem and has convinced the dentist of his or her desire and willingness to change, the second stage can begin. Inevitably, some patients may never move beyond the exploration stage, in which case the educational process should be terminated. As Weinstein (1982) suggests, dentists can and should be selective with whom they work.

In the understanding phase the dentist adopts the role of teacher. Here scientific knowledge and evidence concerning the origins, prognosis, and prevention of dental disease should be presented. The aim is to heighten the patient's awareness of dental disease and to reinforce the views adopted during the exploration phase. The information given to patients should be scientifically valid and any issues which are contentious or ambiguous should be discussed. The advantages and disadvantages of various preventive measures should also be presented.

At this stage the patient's oral care skills should be assessed and training given to remedy any deficiencies observed. Flossing and brushing are technically difficult activities and need to be taught by demonstration and practice.

Once the patient has mastered the required skills it is time to collect baseline data on the patient's home care habits. This is best achieved by giving the patient a chart or diary which can be taped to the bathroom mirror and used to record oral hygiene behaviours. The chart should be designed to provide information on what, when, and for how long particular activities were undertaken. These data allow the dentist to review the patient's current activities and to plan a strategy for change. It also provides a means whereby the patient's progress can be monitored over time.

3 *The action phase*

The collection of baseline data moves the process into the action phase, where behavioural strategies are used to establish new patterns of behaviour. The most detailed account of the use of these strategies in dental practice is to be found in Weinstein *et al.* (1985).

The initial step in the action phase consists of a review of the patient's baseline performance and the setting of realistic intermediate and long-term goals. These goals should be established in consultation with the patient and should be relatively modest. For example, a patient who is brushing once a day may be given the goal of brushing twice a day, or the patient brushing twice a day for 30 seconds should be given the goal of increasing their brushing time to one minute. These relatively modest goals are likely to be achieved by the patient, whereas more ambitious goals might not be achieved and only result in a discouraged individual. Goal setting should be incremental, with additional and equally modest goals only being set once prior goals have been achieved. This continues until optimal levels of oral home care have been established.

The goals that dentist and patient agree are to be set should be detailed and specific rather than general. They should also be written down and given to the patient. Some have found it helpful if these goals are presented in the form of a written contract which is signed by both parties. Such contracts have been found to elicit more cooperation on the part of the patient than agreements which are verbal.

At this stage behavioural techniques which help patients to develop new home care routines can be employed. These can be based on the manipulation of the antecedents or consequences of home care behaviours. Consequences in the form of positive reinforcements of the kind described earlier increase the probability that oral hygiene procedures will continue to the point where they become habit. These can be provided by the dentist, the patient, or the family, and can be material or social in nature. These rewards need to be immediate and continuous if they are to be successful. Patients can be encouraged to award themselves points each time a behaviour is undertaken or a set of goals reached, and then to reward themselves with an activity or acquisition once some overall total is achieved. Family members should also be recruited to reward the individual by means of praise for successful outcomes.

Manipulating the antecedents of behaviour provides the patient with cues which stimulate the patient to brush or floss as required. A chart taped to the bathroom mirror on which all such behaviours are to be recorded serves as a constant and useful reminder. With some patients oral care can be tied to some other already habitual behaviour. Since most people undertake body care activities such as washing and showering on a daily basis, patients should be encouraged to undertake oral care *prior* to these activities. This has the effect of increasing the frequency if not the duration of these behaviours.

Self-monitoring is another important technique that can be used. Charts and records which have to be completed by the patient act as cues and consequences; they stimulate behaviours while providing patients with feedback about progress towards desired goals. Weinstein and colleagues have recently developed a Self-Inspection Plaque Index (SIPI) which patients can use to recognize areas of the mouth which are being inadequately cleaned. This means that patients can monitor not only the frequency of their behaviours but their efficacy in maintaining a high standard of oral hygiene.

During this stage follow-up visits are necessary so that the practitioner can review the patient's home care regimen, identify skill deficiencies or other aspects of the programme which are problematic, and modify the programme if necessary. Goals may need to be renegotiated and contracts rewritten. At these visits the patient should be given encouragement and support, and, whenever possible, shown their achievements to date, using charts or graphs of brushing frequencies, oral hygiene scores, or levels of gingivitis.

4 The habituation phase

Once final goals regarding oral home care have been reached the programme can be terminated. The programme should be withdrawn in stages and arrangements made for periodic review and follow-up. These follow-ups can also serve as booster sessions to remedy any lapses in skill or efficacy. Some degree of regression to old habits should be expected, although these can often be minimized by the use of self-maintenance techniques involving the SIPI.

Clearly, counselling and effective patient education can be time-consuming and labour intensive. They are often a source of frustration for the individual dentist, who may find it difficult to appreciate that patients do not necessarily view dental disorders with the same degree of urgency or importance as the professional. They can also be difficult to implement, since they do not call upon the technical skills in which dentists are highly trained. Moreover, irrespective of the kind of funding system in which the dentist works, either private, public fee for service, or capitation payment, they are unlikely to be financially rewarding. Nevertheless, effective education does means that all phases of the counselling approach need to be used and that the provision of information, however necessary, is insufficient in and of itself.

12

Stress in dental practice

Arguably, dentists are subject to a greater variety of occupationally induced risks to health than any other professional or individual in a health care related occupation. Dentists encounter aerosol hazards in the form of minute particles of tooth structure or dental materials; infectious diseases such as herpes, hepatitis and AIDS; contamination of the work environment by X-rays, mercury, or anaesthetic gases; chemical, thermal, and other injuries; high noise levels; postural problems and physical and psychological stress. Apart from the recent and exaggerated risk of AIDS, it seems that the most lethal of these occupational hazards is stress. Many articles on stress are to be found in the literature aimed at the dental profession and auxiliary occupations, and at least two carry titles such as 'Stress in dentistry — it can kill you' (Lang-Runtz 1984, Lang 1981). One of these articles claims that stress is now the greatest threat to dentists' health and well-being and quotes the following evidence: (1) emotional illness ranks third in order of frequency of health problems among dentists while in the general population it ranks tenth; (2) coronary disease and high blood pressure are over 25 per cent more prevalent among dentists than among the general population; (3) dentists suffer psycho-neurotic disorders at a rate 2.5 times that of physicians; (4) seven out of ten dentists will die of stress-related coronary artery diseases; (5) dentists have the highest rate of suicide of all occupational groups; (6) the suicide rate of dentists is more than twice the rate of the general population and is almost three times higher than that of other white collar workers (Lang 1981). Others have claimed that

There is a growing body of evidence that suggests increased

> vulnerability within the profession to certain disorders and afflictions that can only be categorised as practice-related. The dentist may be subject to a wide variety of physical ailments that are induced or aggravated by the work environment. (Forrest 1978: 361)

The studies on which this characterization of dentistry is based have been criticized on methodological grounds. Nevertheless, it is the case that many nationally- or regionally-based professional associations believe the problem to be a serious one and have created committees or support organizations to minister to dentists with personal, medical, or financial problems which hinder their ability to provide safe and effective care. One of the first was established by the Massachusetts Dental Association, which formed a Committee on Alcoholism and Chemical Dependency; soon after, the California Dental Association established a Hotline Referral Service for its members. The Ontario Dental Association (ODA), like the British Dental Association, has created a Committee for Dentists at Risk designed to aid those practitioners whose ability to practice has been impaired by social or medical problems. According to the ODA, 10 per cent of their members have acute problems of this kind. There is no way of knowing whether these problems have been precipitated by the strains and stresses of dental practice, whether they are the product of practice-related stress and a vulnerable personality type, or whether they would have occurred anyway. After all, some physicians, some lawyers and some architects will be similarly impaired. The rest of this chapter examines the concept of stress and reviews the evidence used to support the claim that dentistry is a particularly stressful endeavour and dangerous to health.

The concept of stress

As indicated in Chapter 2, stress is one of the most commonly used and one of the most ill-defined concepts. Our awareness and understanding of the pervasiveness of stress and its many effects originates in the work of Selye (1974). Selye defined stress as 'The body's non-specific response to any demand placed upon it, whether that demand is pleasant or not.' Stress has three distinct components: (1) a physically or psychologically challenging situation (referred to as a stressor), (2) the individual's perception or interpretation of this situation, and (3) the individual's physiological and psychological responses to the situation. Both (2) and (3) tend to be unique to the individual and influenced by personality traits and other psychological characteristics.

It would be a mistake to assume that stress is necessarily negative in terms of its impact:

> Stress is not something to be avoided; in fact, it cannot be avoided. As the response to a stressor, a stimulus, a set of circumstances that induces a change in the flow of physiological and/or psychological functioning, it's as inevitable and as essential and useful a part of living as changes in breathing and blood circulation produced when exercise is the stressor. Depending upon their intensity and the way they affect the individual, stress reactions can be pleasurable as well as helpful. But when they are inappropriate or excessive, they can exhaust the capacity to respond and lead to difficulty — emotional distress, behavioural disturbances or symptoms of illness. (Selye 1974: 12)

Accordingly, Selye distinguishes between *eustress* which energizes, challenges, develops, and enriches our lives and *distress* which burdens, overwhelms, and debilitates us.

When faced with any kind of stressor the human body responds in a manner which Selye termed the general adaptation syndrome (GAS). Typical changes include a rise in systolic blood pressure and adrenal hormone levels. Long-term stressors cause a collapse of these adaptive mechanisms, a depletion of body defences, and emotional and physical malfunctioning. However, stress and its outcomes are highly variable and one individual will flourish when faced with a given stressor while another will succumb immediately. Some of the main variables which moderate the stress response or its outcomes are the personality of the individual, access to information, past experience and coping skills, the availability of support from family, friends or peers, and the timing of the arrival of the stressor. For example, Kobasa (1979) studied middle- and upper-level executives in American industry and found that only a few experienced problems even though all had high scores when assessed on a life-stress scale. She identified a group of personality factors which characterized these resistant types: (1) *sense of control* — they believed that they controlled the events in their lives and did not feel overwhelmed or powerless in the face of adversity, (2) *sense of commitment* — they were committed to their work and activities, and (3) *sense of challenge* — change was not seen as threatening but as a challenge that aided personal development and growth. Similarly, Brown and Harris (1978) found that women faced with stressful life events were less likely to succumb to depression if they had a supportive relationship with their spouse.

Sources of stress in dental practice

Many articles which have appeared in the popular and scientific literature have commented on the nature of dental practice and identified numerous potential sources of stress. Christen (1984), for example, lists 19 operational, interpersonal, and environmental stressors to which dentists are subjected in the course of their working day (see Table 12.1). Similarly, Forrest (1978) cites professional isolation, physical confinement, high caseloads, economic pressures, the necessity to deal with anxious patients or people in pain, the lack of recognition and appreciation by patients, and the stress of constantly striving for perfection as the most damaging of the stressors associated with dental practice. Forrest (1978) also considers that the personality traits which characterize a good dentist are traits that predispose to depression. He claims that dental schools frequently select candidates with an obsessive–compulsive character, which carries with it a proneness to depression in mid-life, possible drug and alcohol abuse and a risk of suicide.

Ayer and Morretti (1985) have questioned this somewhat alarming characterization of dentists and dental practice. They believe that the stress associated with dental practice has been grossly exaggerated and draw on a body of theory from social psychology to suggest that dentists may be less vulnerable to stress than other occupational groups. For example, dentists have a high degree of control over when, how, and with whom they work and can avoid some of the stress to which they might otherwise be subject. They can eliminate anxious or complaining patients from their practice, modify their hours, or emphasize those aspects of their work they find enjoyable and rewarding. In addition, dentists generally have high incomes and a high socioeconomic status, and so have access to many resources and opportunities, such as decent housing, good medical care, vacations, leisure and exercise, which

Table 12.1 A list of some potentially destructive stressors in dental practice

Operational stressors

- Physical immobility of dental personnel to a fixed office and relatively restricted surrounding working space
- Compulsive attention to cleanliness, orderliness, and perfectionistic details that are inherent in dentistry
- The physical difficulty and mentally taxing nature of dental treatment that must be completed in a restricted, dark, wet oral area
- The necessity of processing patients in a highly structured setting in a clockwork fashion
- Time pressure problems
- Few opportunities to share experiences and relieve stresses through peer support
- Meeting the high costs of equipping an office and coping with overheads as high as 60% of gross income

Interpersonal stressors

- The constant pressure of decision making, plus the continual soothing and counselling of complaining patients
- Anxiety, apprehension, fear, and pain which are frequently present in the dental situation
- Frequent overt verbal rejection by patients
- The necessity to hire and fire personnel
- The necessity to perform in a variety of roles for which the dentist may be ill-prepared, e.g. manager, salesperson, teacher

Office environmental stressors

- Physical fatigue and injuries related to day-to-day practice
- Inadequate lighting
- Excessive sound and noise
- Air pollution from gaseous or particulate materials
- Eye and facial injuries emanating from dental procedures
- Exposure to contagious disease
- Improper control of ionizing radiation

Source: Christen 1984

moderate the effects of any stress they might experience. While Ayer and Morretti concede that dentistry will be stressful for some practitioners, they claim that there is no reason to believe that dental practice is necessarily any more stressful than any other profession.

A number of surveys of dentists have been published which lend support to the view that many dentists find aspects of their work stressful. Unfortunately, only one of these studies was based on a random sample of dentists (Cooper *et al.* 1987); the remainder were small scale and/or used non-representative samples. Howard *et al.* (1976) provide data obtained from 33 Canadian dentists participating in a voluntary fitness clinic, Goodwin *et al.* (1981) surveyed recent graduates from the Michigan school of dentistry, and Cooper *et al.* (1978) and O'Shea *et al.* (1984) asked dentists attending scientific meetings to complete a questionnaire on stress in dentistry. However, despite the differences in their methods, these studies have produced broadly comparable results. The most common sources of stress reported by British dentists are listed in Table 12.2. Many of these, including patient management problems, running behind schedule, interpersonal relations at work, and constraints imposed by third party payers, are not easily controlled by the dentist.

Table 12.2 Most common sources of stress reported by British dentists

Source	Rank
Medical emergency in surgery	1
Difficult, uncooperative patients	2
Running behind schedule	3
Constant time pressures	4
Very nervous patients	5
Dissatisfied patients	6 =
Making mistakes	6 =
High concentration levels	8
Earning enough money for lifestyle needs	9
Patients querying expertise	10 =
Defects in equipment/materials	10 =
Quoting fees and collecting payments	12

Source: Cooper *et al.* 1987

The main drawback with most of these studies is that they identify the most common sources of stress in dental practice but do not provide any information on how *frequently* dentists encounter these problems or the severity of the stress they experience. Dentists do not encounter medical emergencies on a daily basis nor are they necessarily faced with complaining or uncooperative patients during the course of every working day. The one study that provides data on frequency needs to be interpreted with caution since it is based on questionnaires returned by readers of the journal *Dental Economics*, who may not be typical of all dental practitioners (Dunlap and Stewart 1982). Nevertheless, 64 per cent of these dentists reported that they were always or frequently concerned with perfectionism, 56 per cent always or frequently felt under pressure to make more money and 34 per cent always or frequently felt overworked or hurried. They also reported that stress was more severe among dentists who had been in practice for five to fourteen years and more severe in dentists in solo practice. These somewhat pessimistic results need to be viewed in the light of the results of the survey overall. A stress index based on responses to all questions about sources of stress and stress-related symptoms indicated that most of these dentists enjoyed good emotional health and did not seem to be subject to unmanageable stress from multiple sources.

The consequences of stress

Another group of studies has looked at the impact of stress on the individual practitioner. Many of these simply assumed that dentistry was stressful and sought to verify this by examining the mortality and morbidity experience of dental practitioners. The prevalence of suicide among dentists is one potential outcome of high levels of stress which has received particular attention.

Hendrix (1986) has developed a dental stress model which can be used to organize the evidence concerning the impact of stress on the profession (Figure 12.1). He suggests that stress produces physiological and psychological stress responses which have physical and behavioural consequences. Occupational stress can cause a variety of changes in the body (see Chapter 2). These include changes in cholesterol levels, high density lipoproteins, adrenalin, noradrenalin, and triglycerides. At the same time processes such as heart rate, blood pressure, and respiration can all be adversely affected by stress. These may then lead to an increase in the prevalence of disease and premature death.

The psychological responses to stress are an increase in anxiety, depression and irritability and a decrease in job satisfaction and commitment to the job or organization. These result in a reduction in job-related performance, and in absenteeism, habitual lateness, and higher job turnover.

Figure 12.1 Dental stress model based on perceptual job and life stresses

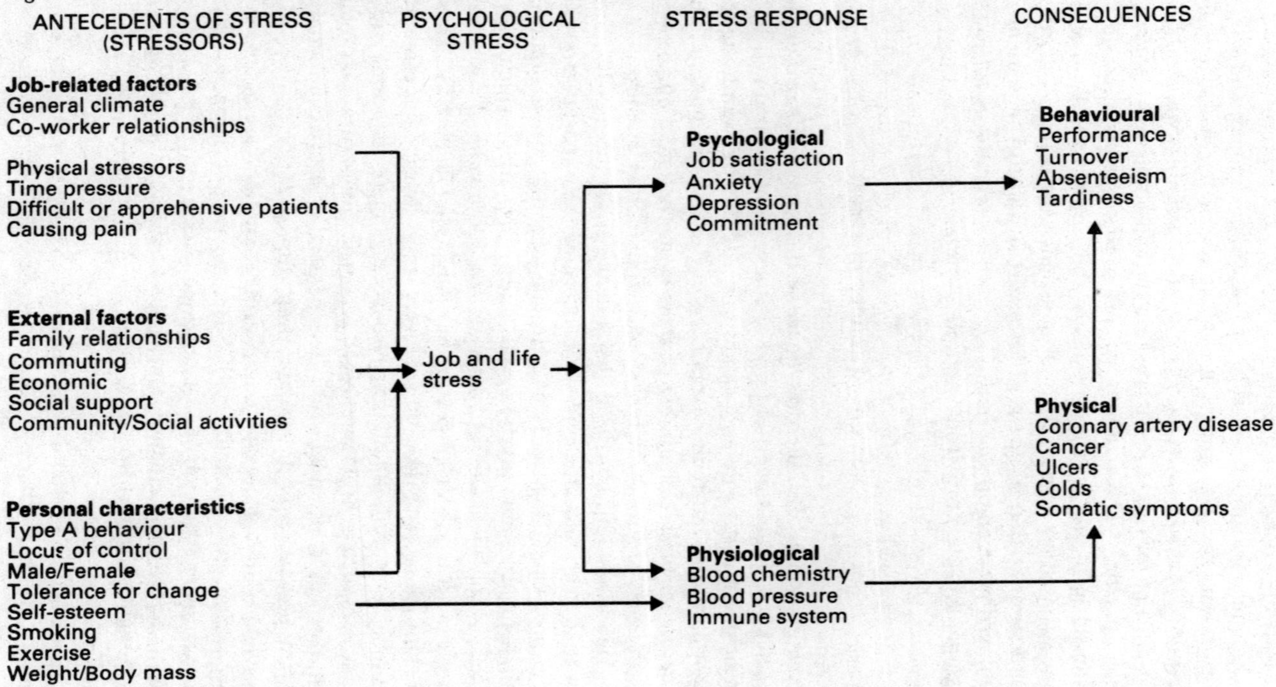

Source: Hendrix 1986

The physical and mental well-being of dentists

One of the earliest studies of the causes of death among dentists was undertaken to determine the frequency with which dentists died of leukaemia as a result of exposure to radiation. Death certificates were examined in order to ascertain cause-specific death rates of dentists who practised in the New England states between 1921 and 1960. The study showed no excess of deaths due to leukaemia and a lower overall death rate than that of the general population. However, the study did show a higher rate of deaths due to suicide (Glass 1966). Subsequent studies of dentists in Oregon, California, and Canada also revealed that dentists had higher suicide rates than did other professional groups and the general population. However, these were based on a small number of deaths in each of the occupations studied and a short time period, and they were confined to a specific geographical area. Consequently, the suicide rates they report may well be unreliable.

A more extensive study was undertaken by Orner (1976), who investigated 102,726 US dentists over a five-year period. Of these, 8,945 were found to have died. The study was unique in that extraordinary efforts were made to determine the vital status of all dentists included in the study and the cause of death of all who had died. It was assumed that differences in mortality for selected causes between dentists and the general population would provide evidence of overexposure to occupational hazards. The study found that approximately 73 per cent of deaths of dentists occurred after the age of 64 years, the overall mortality rate of dentists was lower than that of the population as a whole, and the suicide rate was the same as that of the general population.

The study by Orner is still used to support the claim that dentists are not unduly affected by occupational stress. While this may have been true of the period over which death rates were studied, 1960–5, it is not necessarily the case that the same situation applies today. Over the intervening period dentistry has become more technically complex, patients have become better informed and more demanding, and the financial environment within which dentists work has become more difficult. The impact of these changes on the mortality experience of the profession can only be determined by a new series of studies using more recent and relevant information.

Even if such studies do not show that dentists have higher mortality rates than other professionals or the population as a whole, this provides only limited evidence of the occupational health of the profession. Since mortality rates are an inadequate indicator of health status, other indicators of physical, mental and social well-being need to be taken into account (see Chapter 5). Unfortunately, there is little hard data concerning the physical health of dentists. Early studies found that gastrointestinal disorders, eye-strain, nervous disorders, circulatory problems, and musculo-skeletal disorders were the most common problems reported. However, these studies gave no indication of whether dentists experience an excess of these problems compared to the general population. Dunlap and Stewart (1982) found that many of their respondents admitted to physical and emotional symptoms commonly associated with stress (see Table 12.3), although these rates may be exaggerated owing to the methods used in their study. A recent study of days of work loss due to illness found that general medical practitioners and dentists lost an average of 2.1 and 1.1 days per year respectively. This is much less than the five days of work loss reported by the average worker (Wall *et al.* 1984). However, since dentists are more likely to lose income than the average worker when taking days off, it is not necessarily the case that a lower incidence of work loss means better health among dentists.

Table 12.3 Most common stress symptoms among dentists: percentage reporting that they always or frequently experience the problem

Symptom	%
Feel worried or anxious	38
Feel physically or emotionally exhausted	34
Have headaches and/or backaches	26
Have eating problems	24
Feel irritable or angry	20
Feel depressed	20

Source: Dunlap and Stewart 1982

Some data on the mental health of dentists are provided by a study of general dental practitioners in the UK (Cooper *et al.* 1987). Their sample consisted of 399 males and 85 females aged between their early 20s and late 60s. The survey used a standard index of psychological well-being made up of six sub-scales of mental health: free-floating anxiety, phobic anxiety, obsessionality, somatic anxiety, depression, and hysterical anxiety. The scores obtained from the survey were compared with scores obtained from random samples of the general population. The data showed that male dentists scored significantly higher on four of the six scales than males overall, while female dentists scored significantly higher on two than females as a whole. Cooper *et al.* (1987) believe that the pattern of anxieties revealed are consistent with the high stress factors 'time and income pressures' and 'unfavourable patients' perceptions' also reported in the survey. Part of this they attributed to the changing pattern of funding for dentistry in the UK and the fact that within the NHS patients can change their dentist easily. Whether these anxieties would be typical of dentists working within private free-for-service systems, as in Canada or the US, is not known.

Numerous articles have claimed that practice-related stress in dentistry is responsible for high rates of alcoholism, drug abuse, and divorce among members of the dental profession. Although the US National Council on Alcoholism estimates that the percentage of alcoholics among professionals is one-and-a-half times that among non-professionals, there is very little in the way of hard evidence to support these claims. Studies of medical interns and residents have shown a disturbingly high prevalence of alcohol and drug abuse and marital breakdown but no comparable data exist on the dental profession. One study undertaken in California found that deaths from cirrhosis were no more common among male dentists than the general male population, and a study based on divorce complaints filed in that state found that the rate for dentists was lower than that for the population as a whole and one of the lowest among professionals.

Job dissatisfaction and perceptions of work

Relatively few studies of job satisfaction among dentists have been undertaken, although all have produced similar results. An early study of occupational commitment included dentists, professors, and advertising executives and found that 40 per cent of dentists had low job commitment compared to 16 and 12 per cent respectively for the other occupations (Gerstl 1959). The study concluded that many dentists are committed to their work only to the extent that it is the way in which they make their living. A later study of Welsh dentists asked about their attitudes towards dentistry and found that almost two thirds expressed a liking for their work and only one fifth a dislike. Many complained that the work was tiring and the pace severe, although other factors associated with the work more than compensated for these disadvantages (Eccles and Powell 1967). In a comparable study of pharmacists, Powell and Eccles (1970) found higher rates of satisfaction; 79 per cent of pharmacists enjoyed their work compared to the 60 per cent of dentists expressing satisfaction. The recent survey of dentists in the UK also found that one third expressed considerable dissatisfaction. Most of these were male and over the age of 35 years, a finding consistent with other studies (Cooper *et al.* 1987). Following a review of the literature these authors concluded that this job dissatisfaction rate is two to three times as high as would be expected among professionals.

Whether or not levels of dissatisfaction of this order are associated with the British National Health Service and its method of funding (or underfunding) of dental care is difficult to determine, since no comparable data exist on dentists working within other systems. British dentists are subject to low fees for the services they render, a patient population that may be unable or unwilling to pay privately for care, relatively strict control on clinical decision-making, and, compared to dentists in countries such as Canada, low incomes. The necessity to treat large numbers of patients in order to achieve a level of remuneration consistent with a dentist's professional status may contribute significantly to the problem. It should be noted that 21 per cent of the predominantly US dentists who took part in the survey by Dunlap and Stewart (1982) said that they 'dread going to work', but again there is no guarantee that these are typical of US dentists as a whole. However, it should also be noted that an unpublished study of US dentists found that personality characteristics rather than situational factors influenced the degree of stress experienced and levels of career satisfaction.

According to the model depicted in Figure 12.1, work dissatisfaction may itself have undesirable consequences for job performance or turnover. Of some concern then is whether or not dissatisfied dentists provide a lower or unacceptable standard of technical and/or interpersonal care. Even if quality of care is maintained, dissatisfaction may have a negative impact on practice productivity or efficiency. As yet no studies have investigated these issues nor are there any data on the frequency with which dentists quit dental practice in favour of other careers.

Stress among dental auxiliary staff

The dentist is not the only member of the team providing dental care and not the only member of the team to experience work-related stress. Dental hygienists and assistants also occupy potentially stressful roles and aspects of their working environment likely to generate stress have been identified. A survey of auxiliaries found that they reported the same sources of stress as dentists, experienced similar levels of stress and reported stress-related symptoms almost as frequently (Dunlap and Stewart 1982).

It has been suggested that dental assistants experience more stress than anyone else on the dental team, largely because of their employee status, a lack of control over their work or their time, under-utilization of the skills in which they have been trained, and a lack of participation in the decisions which affect their working lives (Clark and Phillips 1981). According to one study, dental assistants find their work stressful because of its repetitive character, the limited opportunity for career advancement, and the negative attitudes of both dentists and patients. Their low educational and occupational status may mean that they are assigned only relatively menial tasks which, coupled with low levels of remuneration, result in low self-esteem.

Data derived from a detailed study of dental practices in the city of Toronto have identified other, perhaps more important, characteristics of dental assistants' work which may be stressful (Burman 1988). A significant part of their work involves the provision of emotional support to the dentist and the patient. This emotional labour often means that they absorb, and thereby modify, the stress experienced by both, moderating the emotionally charged environment characteristic of dental practice and promoting a more harmonious dentist–patient relationship. The dental assistants interviewed during this study reported that they were more likely to be made aware of patients' fear, anxiety, or dissatisfaction than the dentist, so that managing negative patient affect became their responsibility. In this respect, the function of the dental assistant is akin to that found in other occupational contexts where low status women workers act as mediators between clients and service providers.

From the dentist's point of view, the main problems associated with assistant stress and job dissatisfaction are interpersonal conflict within the dental practice and job turnover. The loss of a staff member disrupts the office routine and causes inconvenience to patients. It also involves a financial loss. Also to be taken into consideration are a lowering of the performance of the person prior to leaving; the direct and indirect costs of advertising, interviewing and recruiting a new person; the time taken to train a new person; and the less than optimal performance of the new person until they have adapted to the job. It has been estimated that the loss of a chairside assistant produces a financial loss of between US$6,000 and US$20,000 at year's end, according to the educational level of the assistant and the time invested in training. Bader (1982) calculated a mean decrease in practice productivity of 16 per cent in the two weeks following the departure of a dental assistant, with a mean decrease of 3 per cent over the longer term.

A number of studies have produced estimates of the magnitude of job turnover among dental assistants, with rates varying from 40 to 83 per cent per annum. The American Association of Dental Assistants has estimated that the rate is between 30 and 40 per cent. A more systematic longitudinal study, albeit of only 13 practices, found that all experienced turnover during a study year, with the rates varying from 13 to 133 per cent. Overall, 26 per cent of the positions in the practices studied experienced turnover and 48 per cent of all auxiliaries left during the course of the year. The difference in the rates indicates that some positions were subject to multiple turnovers (Bader 1982).

Over half the assistants who left the practices included in the study did so for job-related reasons. Most left because of dissatisfaction with remuneration, benefits, status, feedback from the dentist, or a lack of opportunity to influence the office environment or dental care delivery. Given contemporary changes in women's roles, more women are looking for a career rather than a job. Expanding opportunities in other occupational sectors may mean that women are no longer confined to traditionally female occupations but can select from a wider range of careers. There is concern in some quarters that the availability of dental support staff may decline and good staff become exceedingly difficult to find. For example, ADA data show that the number of assistants and hygienists graduating from accredited training programmes has declined. The BDA has also expressed concern at the increasing difficulty faced by dentists in recruiting dental surgery assistants (editorial, *British Dental Journal*). What this means is that the dentist must not only learn how to manage his or her own levels of stress and stress responses, but become adept at managing interpersonal relations in the practice. Principles of organizational behaviour indicate that a participatory rather than an authoritarian management style is necessary to promote staff satisfaction and maintain their membership of the dental team. This kind of team approach is not yet a feature of dental education and may not be easily learned, considering the dentist's training as an isolated operator. Nevertheless, as leader of the dental team it is the dentist's responsibility to seek to improve the pay and career prospects of support staff and to raise their morale by recognizing the value of their work.

Coping with stress

Although the issues of the nature, extent, and consequences of stress in dental practice are not entirely resolved by the data currently at hand, it is clear that some dentists will experience high levels of stress some of the time. That stress may originate in personal crises other than those that are encountered in the work environment or it may involve a combination of life stress and work-related stress. Whatever its origins, such stress needs to be recognized and dealt with. Because stress is so common in the modern day world numerous books and publications are available which describe strategies for managing stress (George *et al.* 1986). These range from self-help techniques to professional counselling for serious personal or career problems. In fact, there are as many ways of managing stress as there are sources of stress and reactions to it.

Selye (1974) identified three antidotes to the stresses of life. These are: learning your own stress levels and organizing your life accordingly, setting your own goals rather than having them imposed upon you, and becoming necessary to other people. George *et al.* (1986) have described physical, environmental, cognitive, and social strategies for stress reduction. Some of these assist the individual to avoid sources of stress. For example, developing a time management system or training in interpersonal skills can help the practitioner to resolve some of the more common sources of stress in dental practice. Others assist the practitioner to transform stress from a negative to a positive experience. This is achieved through a change in attitudes and a change in the way we perceive the events that confront us. Many situations are perceived as threatening even though they pose no real threat. Bringing perceptions more in line with the level of real threat involved reduces the amount of energy required to deal with these stressors. Exaggerated emotional and behavioural response patterns deplete reserves of energy and render an individual even more vulnerable to important life issues (Christen *et al.* 1986).

13

Dentistry as a profession

Dentistry has not always been an organized profession. For much of the eighteenth and nineteenth centuries dental practice was a secondary occupation, undertaken predominantly by tradesmen whose main business might be wigmaking, haircutting, or the selling of medicaments and other 'cures' for physical and psychological disorders. In rural areas, extractions were often performed by blacksmiths or itinerant practitioners who 'performed' at country fairs. For much of this time there was no formal system of dental education and the scientific basis of dentistry was non-existent. From the 1840s onwards, a number of technological developments, such as anaesthesia, X-rays, and amalgam fillings, provided a broader technical basis for dental practice and increased the range of procedures performed in dentistry, but its practitioners remained, with notable exceptions, artisans of relatively low social status.

Associations of dental practitioners were formed around the middle of the nineteenth century, when the first schools for the teaching of dentistry were established in London. In England, where dentistry emerged as a profession somewhat later than it did in Canada and the US, most dentists continued to receive their training by means of an apprenticeship with an established practitioner. Until 1918, only a minority of dentists had received some formal education and a recognized qualification. This situation changed during the 1920s, when legal restrictions were placed on the practice of dentistry, and education and qualification became mandatory. The fortunes of dentistry changed dramatically, so that by the 1950s the dentist was a member of a respected and prestigious profession (Davis 1980). In this regard, organized dentistry was the outcome of a historical process which, more than 50 years earlier in Britain, had given rise to the medical profession.

What is a profession?

Almost everyone would agree that the professions are distinct in some respects from other occupations, but many would be hard pressed to specify the nature and scope of these differences. This might be because the word 'professional' is not limited to dentists, doctors, or lawyers, but is also used to describe sportsmen and women, those who practise the dramatic or sexual arts, and even hardened criminals (Moline 1986). In the case of sportsmen and women, the word is used to identify those who are paid and earn a living from activities others undertake in the pursuit of leisure. In the case of the actor or criminal, it seems to imply a certain standard of conduct while working or a dedication and commitment to a way of life. While financial remuneration, standards of professional practice, and dedication to the job are characteristic of professionals, they are not the only, nor the most important, traits which distinguish dentists and doctors from others who work in health care.

In very general terms all professions have specialized skills which are provided as personal services to clients (Blane 1986). Clearly, this definition is too broad for our purposes, for it would equally apply to many if not most of the occupations involved in the provision of health care, particularly those which have direct contact with patients. For example, it would apply to hygienists as well as dentists, in spite of the other significant differences between them. In an attempt to develop definitions which were more precise, a number of sociologists interested in work and the division of labour attempted to identify the essential features of occupations universally considered to be professions. In undertaking this task they have generally used the medical profession as a model. The most comprehensive list has been produced by Goode (1960), who identified ten key traits characteristic of the professions.

1 A profession determines its own standards of education and training.

2 The professional goes through an extensive period of

education and training in order to acquire highly specialized knowledge and skills.

3 Professional practice requires a licence issued by a legally recognized professional organization.

4 Organizations which license and thereby admit persons to the professions are run by members of the profession itself.

5 The scope of legislation which defines the privileges and obligations of the profession is largely determined by the profession.

6 Members of the profession command high incomes, prestige, and power.

7 The professional practitioner is free from evaluation and control by lay persons.

8 The profession establishes standards of practice and personal conduct, and may revoke the licence of persons not meeting those standards.

9 Members of the profession have a strong identification and affiliation with their professional group.

10 The profession is one to which most members make a lifetime commitment and few leave the profession once they have gained admission to it.

The only characteristics not listed by Goode, but considered important by others who have produced similar lists, are a community orientation and a service ethic. That is, professional training instils in the individual a degree of altruism, whereby serving the community and acting in the best interests of the client are valued more highly than the opportunities for personal gain by professional practice.

There are two main problems with these trait definitions of professions. The first is that many of the characteristics identified would apply to many occupations which are not traditionally accepted as professions and do not have either the status or the power enjoyed by dentistry and medicine. In order to cope with this criticism some have argued that it is difficult, if not impossible, to draw a strict dividing line between the professions and other occupations. They suggest that a more appropriate characterization is a continuum on which all occupations can be ranked as more or less professional. Blane (1986), for example, draws a distinction between the 'leading professions' and the 'lesser professions'. Examples drawn from the health care sector would be medicine and nursing. The former has its own specialized body of knowledge which is continually expanding as a result of research and clinical experience, while the latter's theoretical basis is still, despite an expansion in clinical nursing research, largely derived from that of the former. While both have a certain autonomy in deciding how their work should be done and in determining standards of practice, nurses gain access to their clients only through the instructions of doctors. In fact, the lesser professions were established on the assumption that they would assist the leading professions and undertake the less prestigious patient care activities. Clearly, the same applies to dentists and hygienists. It should come as no surprise that when these professional relationships were established, members of the leading professions were drawn from males of high social status, while the lesser professions were occupied by women of lower social status. To a large extent, these same conditions apply today.

A second problem with this 'essential attributes' approach to the professions is what it implies with regard to professionalization. Here 'professionalization' refers to the historical process by which an occupation is transformed into a profession. According to Wilensky (1964), the emergence of a profession is the result of a logical sequence of events whereby an occupation progressively acquires the defining characteristics listed above and becomes accepted as such by the government of the day and society at large. This progressive professionalization of an occupation consists of five key stages: (1) the emergence of a full time occupation, (2) the founding of a training school, (3) the establishment of a professional association, (4) political agitation to obtain recognition of the profession and its association in law, and (5) the adoption of a code of conduct and professional practice. Unfortunately, historical study shows that there is great variation in the process whereby an occupation becomes a profession, and there is no natural or logical sequence to the process. In addition, the experience of occupations currently in the process of professionalization suggests that the privileges and advantages of becoming a profession, such as high levels of remuneration and the right to practise without outside supervision, do not automatically flow from the acquisition of most of those characteristics which supposedly define a profession. Nursing, for example, remains a lesser or subordinate profession in spite of longer periods of training, the increasing tendency for nurses to be university-trained, and the development of independent nursing research which has begun to provide a scientific and theoretical basis for nursing practice.

A more critical and, it is claimed, historically accurate view of the professions is presented by Freidson (1970) and Johnson (1972). Both agree that the main characteristic which distinguishes the professions from other occupations is that of power and influence. This power has nothing to do with the objective character of the work undertaken by the professions, or the character of the knowledge and training on which that work is based. Rather, professions such as dentistry and medicine emerged out of an essentially political process in which they gained a *monopoly* over a specific field of practice and the right to self-determination and *autonomy*.

The monopoly and autonomy enjoyed by the professions is granted by the state and enshrined in law. In turn, this legally based power gives the profession the exclusive right to provide a personal service such as health care, and establishes its position of authority with regard to the other occupations providing similar or related services. These other occupations, or 'lesser professions', can only practise under the guidance and supervision of a professional. In addition, the profession, by way of its professional organizations and licensing bodies, controls recruitment, education, and practice and is the only body which can judge the performance of its members and discipline them for breaches of professional conduct. In this way, a profession represents a particular form of occupational control. It determines who does its work and how that work shall be done. While other occupations are attempting to attain these privileges, only the professions have been granted the right to exercise them legitimately.

Freidson (1970) considers that a crucial factor in determining whether or not an occupation is granted a monopoly over a personal service and autonomy of practice is the protection and patronage of the political elite who have been persuaded of the special character and value of that occupation's work. The fact that some occupations share some of the characteristics of medicine, dentistry, and the law is used by members of these occupations to justify their claims to professional status and legal recognition. However, in striving to develop a theoretical knowledge base and extended periods of training, some of these professionalizing occupations, such as nursing and social work, have forgotten that medicine attained legal protection at a time when its knowledge base was hardly more scientific than that of the 'unqualified' folk healers it was able to exclude from health care practice.

Freidson's comments seem to imply that an occupation becomes a profession as a result of political action: it convinces the state of the merits of its case and is granted monopoly and autonomy. According to Johnson (1972), the emergence of a profession is a historically specific process which some occupations have undergone at a given point in time, rather than a process which many occupations may be expected to undergo because of their essential qualities. It is no accident that the leading professions, those with a legally protected monopoly and autonomy, emerged during the mid to late nineteenth and early twentieth centuries. This was a time of rapid social and economic change, and a time of great optimism with regard to science and technology, and the potential for humanity to exert control over nature.

Conditions which favoured the development of professions in the second half of the nineteenth century were the growth in the population and the rise of an affluent middle class. This provided a market for personal services, allowed health care to become a full-time occupation, and ended the dependence of the health care elite, the formally educated or trained physicians and dentists, on the patronage of the aristocracy. A second condition favouring the development of autonomy concerns the changing nature of the product provided by the health care occupations. Prior to the mid-nineteenth century, medical practice was based on a range of theories of which none was demonstrably superior to others. This changed with the development of the scientific approach.

Larson (1978) has described the contribution of science to the development of the medical profession. The growing scientific basis of medicine allowed the nascent profession to claim a superiority of approach which, in turn, allowed it to gain credibility in the eyes of both the state and the consulting public. At the same time, a competence gap opened up between the doctor and the patient such that the latter became increasingly dependent upon the former. The specialized body of knowledge to which doctors and dentists had increasing access meant that they, rather than the patient, came to define both the patient's needs and the manner in which they were to be met. This power differential between the doctor and patient, the potential harm that might be involved in medical treatment, and the potential for exploitation of the patient, made necessary some degree of regulation to ensure uniform standards of training and competence in professional practice and a high standard of ethical conduct. The passing of the Medical Registration Act in the UK in 1858 provided the public with a means to distinguish the qualified from the unqualified health care provider. These same conditions also applied to dentistry and favoured the development of an autonomous profession. According to Johnson (1972), attempts by other occupations providing specialized personal services to clients to gain a similar degree of monopoly and autonomy are unlikely to succeed today, partly because of the resistance of the established professions whose interests and dominance may be threatened, but also because the historical conditions facilitating professionalization no longer apply.

The role of professions in modern societies

It should be clear from the above account that the professionalization of medicine and dentistry serves two broad interests. On the one hand, it protects the profession from competition in the market-place and from the scrutiny of outsiders. On the other, it offers some protection to those in need of health care by ensuring a certain standard of clinical competence. Broadly speaking, writers who have attempted to describe the role of professions in modern societies have chosen to emphasize either the interests of the patient and the community at large, the self-interests of the leading professions, or the interests of the economic and political elite in society.

One view of the professions is derived from a theoretical tradition called 'functionalism'. Simply put, this approach explains the existence of social institutions, organizations, and patterns of behaviour in terms of their contribution to the smooth operation of society and its long-term stability. Accordingly, the professions perform vital functions without which the fabric of society would, it is claimed, collapse. The health care professions developed in response to the need of societies to minimize and control illness, a major impediment to the ability of the individual to undertake major social roles such as work and parenting. The control of illness required the emergence of a coherent group who would use highly specialized, technical knowledge in pursuit of this essential function. Because the concentration of scientific knowledge in the hands of such a group would make the community vulnerable to exploitation, the training of health care professionals and their socialization into the professional role impart the values of altruism and service to the community. In return, society grants exclusive control of health and illness to the professions and rewards them by high status and high incomes (Parsons 1951).

According to the functionalist view, the dependency and vulnerability of the sick mean that health care cannot be provided within the mechanism of an open market in which almost anyone can offer to provide health care. Rather, it must be the exclusive preserve of a group who are demonstrably superior in terms of technical expertise and moral character. A more critical approach has been adopted by other theorists who are less convinced of the benevolence of the professions. Freidson, who is largely concerned with analyzing the role of the medical profession, claims that the main aim of a profession is to serve its own interests and maintain its position of dominance, power, and prestige. Evidence that the health care professions are more concerned with their own interests rather than those of the community might be found in their sometimes vigorous opposition to the funding of health care by the state — a funding which would remove the economic barriers to health care otherwise encountered by many in the middle and lower income groups — and their opposition to payment mechanisms such as capitation, which seek to control costs. According to Freidson, the community orientation and altruism of the medical profession are more apparent than real, and are simply ideological devices which assist the profession to maintain its exclusive position in the medical market-place. Paradoxically, this view is shared by Milton Friedman, an economist, who also believes these claims are fraudulent. The resulting professional monopoly of health care makes its provision inefficient. A profession's right to control not only the content of professional training but also the numbers trained means it can manipulate the supply of its services and protect its scarcity value and its income.

Other commentators have given more emphasis to the ways in which the professions influence not only the institutions within which they work but also the community at large. Using medicine as an example, they point out that medical practice not only controls illness but acts as an agency of *social* control (Zola 1975). This is evident in the necessity for the sick to have their sickness legitimated by a doctor; that is, people cannot simply claim that they are ill and abandon their social responsibilities. Ultimately, employers and the welfare system require that this is officially sanctioned by a doctor. In this way the doctor acts as a gatekeeper to the sick role and ensures that individuals who are fit and healthy remain active in the workforce and society at large.

A related but broader criticism has been directed at the practice of psychiatry. Szasz (1961) claims that mental illness is not an objective disorder in the same way that physical illness is. It constitutes a convenient label and a way of dealing with people whose behaviour, thoughts, and feelings are socially disruptive. Psychiatric diagnoses are not medical judgements based on observable or detectable organic malfunction, but social and political judgements about the appropriateness of behaviour. Zola (1975) believes that there is an increasing tendency in modern societies for moral and ethical issues to be defined as medical problems and brought under the control of the medical profession. This process, referred to as 'medicalization', means that the medical profession becomes a major player in the social conflict over issues such as abortion and euthanasia. Not everyone has viewed this development in a negative way. Some argue that it is better for alcoholics and drug addicts to be defined as ill and in need of treatment rather than as moral degenerates and deserving of punishment.

A final criticism of the professions in society comes from those who subscribe to a Marxist approach to social analysis. Simply put, this attempts to demonstrate the ways in which social institutions or organizations serve the interests of the economic and political elite in society — the so called 'ruling class'. Again, medicine has been a major target of this critique.

According to the Marxist critique, the ruling class is distinguished by its ownership of the means by which wealth is produced, the endless drive to extract profit from the work force, and its dominance of the political system by means of which its economic position and power are protected. Writers such as McKinlay (1977) and Navarro (1976) claim that medicine aids this process in a number of ways.

First, health is itself a commodity to be bought and sold, and health care is a major and highly profitable industry. The pharmaceutical industry, insurance companies which provide coverage for health care, and the owners of private hospitals all benefit in this way. McKinlay claims that the potential of medicine to generate profit means that health care is not distributed according to need but according to the need to maximize profit. The vulnerability of patients can be exploited in terms of their need to buy health care from a closed market. Second, medicine improves and maintains the health of the workforce and promotes the productive capacity of labour; and third, medicine hides the real nature and causes of ill health. According to Navarro, medicine individualizes health problems, viewing them as failures in biology. This masks the real environmental and occupational causes of disease which, if widely known, would result in pressure for social change.

Most of these criticisms of professional organizations have been directed at medicine rather than dentistry largely because medical practitioners have a broader field of operation and greater involvement in the lives of their patients. Nevertheless, many could equally be applied to the dental profession. So which of these views is correct and in whose interests do the health professions act? It is difficult to give a generalized answer since all of these views contain elements of truth and all contain views which are manifestly wrong (Hart 1985). For example, there is no contradiction in claiming that most dentists act in the best interests of their patients, providing treatment that is or is believed to be appropriate for the patient's condition, but that the profession as a whole acts to protect its own interests when its monopoly and autonomy are threatened. At the same time, the profession may promote the interests of the community by political action designed to instigate preventive procedures such as fluoridation or to persuade food manufacturers to reduce the sugar content of their products. The wide range of interests the profession protects and pursues is to be expected, given the broader context of a complex and highly developed society.

Threats to professionalism

If professionalism is defined in terms of monopoly and autonomy then a number of challenges to professionalism have emerged since the 1960s. One such challenge is to be found in critiques of the effectiveness of modern medicine and its scientific basis, and the argument, largely derived from the work of McKeown (see Chapter 1), that health is socially and environmentally determined and does not flow from clinical practice and medical intervention based on high technology. These critiques are reviewed in Chapter 15. Another potential challenge is to be found in the attempts of many auxiliary occupations in both medicine and dentistry to seek organizational independence from leading professions and/or the right to independent practice.

As a response to the increasing complexity of medical practice, both dentistry and medicine have delegated some tasks to auxiliaries. In the case of dentistry, these have been technicians, dental, assistants, dental therapists and dental hygienists. The training and the work of auxiliary staff is largely determined and directed by the dental profession. In most instances, auxiliary staff who provide treatment services must work under the prescription of a supervising dentist who retains responsibility for diagnosis and treatment planning, and the overall care of the patient. In a few circumstances, such auxiliaries have obtained limited rights to independent practice. This tends to happen in situations of high need and low supply of professionals. In New Zealand, for example, dental nurses have been working in schools since 1923. They may diagnose and provide a limited range of treatments for schoolchildren, including the use of local anaesthesia and the extraction of deciduous teeth. However, their services are confined to children and they may only work in the Public Health Dental Service. Although they are under the supervision of a dentist, the dentist does not have to be on the premises while they provide treatment. The dentist is, however, responsible for ensuring that the nurse is providing effective dental care. Dental therapists also work in the remote northern communities of Canada providing services to native peoples.

Where these types of auxiliaries do not directly threaten the market serviced by dentists they tend to be tolerated by organized dentistry. The same does not apply to denturists: former dental technicians who have obtained the right to provide full and, in some cases, partial dentures. Denturists are allowed to practise in parts of the US, Canada, Australia, Switzerland, and Finland, although the regulations governing their practice vary considerably. In Ontario, denturists can offer a full denture service, including all the clinical and technical stages involved, without the supervision of a dentist, and they may provide partial dentures under the supervision of a dentist. Technicians obtained these rights following a highly organized political campaign. They were successful in spite of the vigorous opposition of the dental profession to this infringement of their market. Currently, Ontario denturists are seeking to expand their independent practice to include partial dentures. As well as challenging the monopoly of the profession, denturists tend to reinforce the view that dentistry is essentially a technical rather than a scientifically based clinical endeavour and, from the perspective of the dental profession, undermine its status and prestige. The pay-off to the community is a low cost denture service. More recently, hygienists in Ontario have been granted organizational autonomy, an autonomy opposed by the dental profession, which used to control dental hygiene through the Royal College of Dental Surgeons. Some have argued that licensing hygienists to practice independently is the answer to the problem of providing oral health care to the homebound and the institutionalized elderly.

A more potent threat to the autonomy of the health care professions is to be found in attempts to control the costs of general and dental health care. Third-party payers, in the form of governments or insurance companies, are attempting to contain costs by the development of new payment mechanisms and new forms of health care organization, some of which have been greeted with a conspicuous lack of enthusiasm by the health care professions. Most clearly under threat is the practitioner's clinical freedom. Medical decision-making is increasingly under review from within and outside the profession. This has been stimulated by the concerns of consumers for high quality care and by third-party payers who are anxious for health care professionals to take account of the economic implications of their clinical decision-making. Certainly, the health care professions of the future will have to work within a social and economic environment far removed from that enjoyed by their predecessors.

For example, a major strategy for containing the cost of hospital care in the US is the shift from payment on a fee-for-service basis to one based on Diagnosis-Related Groups (DRGs). Under this system, hospitals are paid a fixed sum for each patient admitted, based on factors such as the patient's diagnosis and age. Because the hospital is no longer paid for each item of service rendered, it is possible to make a financial loss in treating a patient. One consequence of this is that hospitals keep accurate financial records and send practice and financial profiles to doctors or nursing teams which clearly identify who is ordering more tests or using more expensive treatments than average. Health care professionals may then be called upon to justify their mode of medical practice. Some professionals believe this will compromise the quality of the care given and make clinical practice subordinate to the economic goals of hospital finance officers. Capitation schemes and Health

Maintenance Organizations, increasingly favoured under both state and private systems of health care financing, also involve economic constraints and incentives with regard to clinical decision-making (see Chapter 14).

Other consequences of cost containment are not so much a threat to professionalism but to the dental profession itself. Although frequently opposed by health professionals, state funding of health care through taxation or compulsory insurance schemes have benefitted the professions by broadening the market for their services. Private health insurance schemes have had the same effect. However, in an effort to contain costs, some of the burden of payment is, or is likely, to be shifted back to the patient. Under the British system, non-exempt patients only receive free dental care when the costs of that care rise above a certain level. It has recently been proposed that patients should pay for the initial examination, an aspect of the service traditionally covered by the state. Similarly, private insurers can reduce their payments by cost-sharing mechanisms such as deductibles and co-payment. Such measures depress the demand for dental health care and may ultimately threaten the economic well-being of the profession.

The extent to which these changes in the environment of professional health care practice challenge the autonomy and monopoly of dentistry or medicine has been a matter of debate. Haug (1975) has characterized the current period as one of 'deprofessionalization'. Freidson (1986) believes this exaggerates the challenge to the professions, for the legal position of dentists and doctors, the source of their strength and power, remains unchanged and will do so in the foreseeable future.

14
The organization of dental health care

All industrialized countries have some form of organized health care system of which dentistry is a part. These systems are similar to the extent that medical and dental care is undertaken by fundamentally different types of providers and there is a basic distinction between primary care and hospital care. In other respects, however, the systems differ markedly. There are differences in structure, methods of financing, and methods of paying providers, as well as differences in the types of personnel who provide dental care.

A distinction is often drawn between the private or 'free market' health care system of the US and the 'socialized' or publicly financed system of the UK. Canada, which relies on a system of compulsory, publicly administered insurance, and the European countries, which are financed by combinations of general taxation and public and private insurance schemes, are seen to fall somewhere in between.

These characterizations do not do justice to the complexity of the systems to which they refer. Both the US and the UK, for example, have mixed systems in which public and private provision coexist. Although the British National Health Service is financed largely through general taxation, patient fees are becoming a more important part of the system. This is particularly the case with dentistry, where patients who are not exempt from charges, such as children, the poor, and the low-income elderly, are required to pay out of pocket for part of the cost of a course of treatment. These fees are increasing over time and covering an increasing range of services provided by the dentist, a trend that has been referred to as the 'privatization' of dental care (Birch 1985).

Changes in the system of levying patient contributions, which became effective in 1985, increased the proportion of dental treatment costs borne by the patient to 67 per cent (Nuttall 1985). At the same time, a small and growing private health care system exists alongside the NHS. Both doctors and dentists can practise within the NHS and also take private patients who pay fees or are covered by private health insurance. Similarly, although the US system is predominantly a private one, over 40 per cent of the cost of health care is financed through taxation. Medicare and Medicaid schemes pay for care for the elderly and the poor who fall outside the system of private health care insurance. In Canada, medical care is financed through a health insurance scheme but there is little in the way of a private medical care system. Private insurance schemes to pay for medical care are not allowed by law. Dentistry, however, falls largely in the private sector, although most provinces have publicly funded programmes for children and those on welfare, and one, Alberta, has a programme for the elderly. A substantial proportion of the working population is covered by occupationally linked dental insurance schemes which pay all or most of the cost of care for the insured and their dependants.

Private and public provision of dental health care

Differences in the way health care systems are organized and financed are the product of differences in prevailing social and political philosophies, the relative power of vested interests such as those of consumers and health care professionals, and responses to short-term political pressures or longer-term social realities. The earliest example of state intervention in health care happened in Germany in the 1880s. The state-sponsored health insurance scheme introduced by Bismarck was not a humanitarian gesture in the name of health, but part of a political strategy to halt the spread of socialist ideas and limit the influence of socialist political parties among German workers.

The above factors, combined with newer concerns about the cost and efficiency of health care, ensure that health care systems are in a constant state of evolution. The changes thus entailed may be perceived by the powerful health care professions as undermining their self-interest and may be strongly resisted, although, in the case of dentistry, this resistance may be somewhat tempered by concerns about the shrinking of the traditional market for dental care (see Chapter 1). Under these circumstances, public provision for the care of previously under-serviced groups and currently unattractive methods of financing may become acceptable as solutions to the much discussed problem of a decline in the 'busyness' of dental practices.

One of the fundamental conflicts in health policy has been between those who favour a free market system and those who believe that health should be publicly financed and free at the point of delivery. Although no health care system conforms to these models, it is worth considering the arguments for and against them.

Many of those who believe in a free market for health care base this belief on philosophical views about the nature of human beings and society, and political ideas regarding the legitimate role of governments in providing for the needs of the population. Where health professionals adhere to the idea of a free market, they are more likely to be committed to fee-for-service private practice based on free choice and the absence of external constraints imposed by third-party payers such as governments. The main advantages for the professional which flow from this traditional method of delivering health care are those of flexibility and choice. Patients are able to choose their dentist and dentists are able to choose which patients they will and will not treat. Moreover, the only constraints on the volume and nature of services provided are the patient's ability and willingness to pay. According to this view, private practice is believed to be the most efficient way of delivering dental care, to maximize productivity and quality, and to ensure the clinical freedom of the practitioner.

Many of these features are, of course, characteristic of dental practice within dental care systems which are publicly financed. The majority of dentists in Britain are private practitioners who contract with the NHS to provide services to patients. The main disadvantage of this system from the dentist's perspective is that a set fee is paid for each procedure and it cannot be varied according to the patient's ability to pay. Nor does it necessarily reflect the quality of the work done or the experience of the dentist undertaking the procedure.

A supposedly free market system also has advantages and disadvantages for patients and society as a whole. The main advantage of a system in which patients buy health care is that the demand for care is limited by price. Once prices begin to outstrip the patient's ability to pay, then the use of health services declines. The market mechanism is such that supply and demand achieve an equilibrium so that governments do not have the responsibility of assessing health care needs and determining the volume of service needed to meet them.

Clearly, a free market system in which health care is treated like any other commodity does not and cannot exist. Patients are not free to choose health care in the same way in which they are free to choose clothing or consumer durables. One of the reasons for this is that patients are insufficiently knowledgeable about their health care needs and how they are best met. The market for health care also violates most of the other principles of free markets. First, the health professions monopolize the provision of health care and legal restrictions prevent alternative providers offering similar services to consumers. Second, professional restrictions on advertising mean that there is little in the way of direct competition between providers and it is rarely possible for a patient to shop around for the best deal. Finally, the producer makes the decision regarding the volume and nature of the service provided, so that price is not a very effective regulatory mechanism.

However, the main problem with the free market is that health care is limited to those that can afford to pay, even though the greatest need for health care is to be found among those who are the least likely to have the resources to buy it. Private insurance schemes are one solution to this problem but do not offer universal coverage and generally miss uninsurable groups such as the elderly, the chronic sick, and the unemployed. Consequently, governments are obliged to step in to remedy the failings of the free market.

The main characteristic of a publicly funded system of health care is that demand is more closely related to need and independent of the ability to pay. Although removal of the economic barrier to the use of health services can mean that overall expenditures tend to rise, the supposed benefits are a more equitable distribution of services and, ultimately, a healthier population. This was the assumption underlying the creation of the NHS in Britain, although experience has shown that inequalities in both health and health service use not only continue to exist but may have widened over time.

The main problem with a publicly funded health care system is that of meeting demand within finite resources. In such a system, mechanisms other than price have to be devised to ration health care. One option is to set a ceiling on the resources allocated to health care so that demand over and above what these resources can provide results in queues and waiting lists. Governments also become involved in complex decisions regarding the allocation of resources both regionally and between different areas of health need. However, by setting overall limits on health care spending it becomes easier to control the rising costs of health care. Britain, for example, spends far less of its Gross National Product on health than the US, with its more market-oriented system.

Dental insurance and its effects

The dental insurance schemes which provide cover for an increasing proportion of the North American population modify the 'free market' system of provision by reducing the financial impact of dental care. Properly speaking, they are not a form of insurance but are third-party prepayment plans. The third party in this case is usually a private insurance company which administers the plan with the aim of generating a profit, or a non-profit-making private or public body. Generally, insurance consists of a group of unconnected individuals paying premiums at regular intervals to compensate any subscribing individual for a catastrophic loss. Prepayment, however, is a mechanism for spreading the costs of dental care over a group. Here monthly premiums are paid wholly by an employer or jointly by an employer and his or her employees to an insurer or policy carrier in order to provide coverage for an identifiable group such as the members of a trade union or professional association (Burt 1983). Because private dental insurance schemes generally cover groups and not individuals they are usually obtained as an occupationally linked benefit. Individual policies are available, but characterized by high premiums and a limited coverage of services.

By offering dental insurance plans to groups rather than individuals, insurance companies are able to make sure that they include people with low as well as high dental care needs. In effect, the former subsidize the latter and enable the plan to remain profitable. In addition, a number of other mechanisms have been used to reduce the amount of benefits paid by the carrier on behalf of the insured. These include: (1) limiting the range of services covered by the plan, (2) having the patient pay part of the cost in the form of a deductible, (3) having the patient pay part of the cost by co-insurance, (4) building in a waiting period after joining the plan before any benefits are paid, (5) setting annual expenditure limits per patient, and (6) requiring pre-authorization for courses of treatment which cost more than a stipulated sum. In plans which contain a deductible, the insurance carrier pays the costs of dental care only if they exceed a stipulated, and usually nominal, amount. In the case of co-insurance the patient pays a stipulated percentage of the cost of dental care.

Most private insurance carriers reimburse dentists on a fee-for-service basis, although payment by capitation has become increasingly attractive as a means of limiting dental health care expenditures. Unlike insurance schemes run by non-profit corporations, such as the Delta Dental Plans in the US, or the publicly funded system of the British NHS, private insurance carriers do not require that post-treatment examinations of samples of patients are undertaken by independent dentists to ensure that work for which fees were claimed has been done and is of an acceptable quality. Nevertheless, some dentists, as with some doctors, regard the third-party payer, whether a commercial company, non-profit corporation or the state, as compromising the sanctity of the patient–practitioner relationship. Consequently, where market conditions permit, some health care professionals wish, and are able, to opt out of some schemes.

Third-party payment plans have grown phenomenally since their inception in the 1960s and 1970s. In 1970, less than one per cent of the population of Ontario was covered by dental insurance. By 1979, this had risen to 43 per cent. Similar increases have been observed in the US and it is likely that dental insurance will become a feature of the British dental care system as increasing emphasis is placed by governments on the private health care sector. This growth in coverage is due to the desire of trade unions or professional associations to extend the health-related benefits provided by employers and the willingness of insurers to provide plans on a group basis. Neither of these groups is motivated by broad social policy issues such as reducing inequalities in access to dental care by removing economic barriers. This was a major aim of the British National Health Service and Canada's medical care insurance systems. Nevertheless, health insurance in general and dental health insurance in particular have been major areas of policy debate. Some have argued that public provision, or state or privately sponsored insurance schemes, whereby care is provided free at the point of delivery, bring about a more equitable distribution of health services and are of particular benefit to low-income families. Others have argued that the removal of the price barrier to health care leads to unrestricted and inappropriate use of services and rising costs.

Until recently, little was known about the effect of insurance or the provision of free care on the use and costs of dental services. Although many studies have been undertaken since the 1960s, most are weak methodologically and unable to sort out the effects of insurance from the effects of other predisposing and enabling variables. The Rand Health Insurance Study (Manning *et al.*1986), however, used an experimental design in order to assess the effect of insurance and different cost-sharing arrangements on the utilization of dental care by comparable groups of people.

Families from six sites in the US were randomly selected and randomly assigned to one of several fee-for-service health insurance plans with different co-insurance rates. The percentage of costs paid out of pocket were 0 per cent (i.e. free), 25 per cent, 50 per cent and 95 per cent respectively. Each of these plans had an upper limit of 5, 10 or 15 per cent of family income up to a maximum of $1000. This meant that once family expenditure on *all* health care exceeded this limit all costs were paid in full. An individual deductible plan was also included but it is not described here. Utilization data for families enrolled in these plans were obtained directly from claims filed by the participants. This included the percentage visiting the dentist in the previous year, the number of visits per year, and the type and costs of services consumed.

Because there was an initial surge in demand during the first year of the experiment the effects of different levels of insurance were estimated using data from the second or 'steady-state' year. In the analysis the plan in which patients paid for 95 per cent of the costs of dental care is treated as the control since this group approximates a non-insured group. The results are given in Tables 14.1 and 14.2.

Utilization increased significantly as the cost of care to the patient fell. The probability of any use of dental services during the steady-state year was 31 per cent higher for those on the free compared to those on the 95 per cent co-insurance plan. In addition, those receiving free care had 34 per cent more visits and expenditures that were 46 per cent higher than those enrolled in the 95 per cent plan. The 50 and 25 per cent co-insurance plans had small and insignificant effects on utilization when compared with the 95 per cent plan.

Table 14.1 Rand Health Insurance Study: predicted annual steady-state use of dental services by insurance plan

Plan	Probability of any use (%)	Mean visits per person	Mean costs per person
Free	66.1	1.87	$243
25%	52.3	1.47	$185
50%	49.8	1.41	$165
95%	50.5	1.40	$166

Source: Manning *et al.* 1986

Table 14.2 Percentage changes in utilization: all plans v. *95 per cent plan*

	Probability of any use	Visits per enrollee	Expenditures per enrollee
Free *v.* 95%	+ 31	+ 34	+ 46
25% *v.* 95%	+ 4	+ 5	+ 11
50% *v.* 95%	− 1	+ .7	+ .6

Source: Calculated from the data provided by Manning *et al.* 1986

Analysis of the data by income showed that free care increased the probability of use and the number of visits by 45 and 46 per cent respectively for those with low incomes and by 22 and 26 per cent respectively for those with high incomes when compared with their respective controls. As expected, low income groups were more price sensitive; that is, as the direct costs of dental care increased their use of dental services decreased more sharply than that of wealthier individuals.

Containing the costs of dental care

In all industrialized countries health care costs have increased alarmingly. This is particularly the case in the US, where a number of mechanisms have been instituted in an attempt to keep costs under control. Health care costs in Britain have largely been controlled by budgetary restraint and it is likely that fundamental changes in financing and organization will take place in the future to promote the efficiency of the system and further constrain public expenditures.

Data from the US show that dental care costs have risen more slowly than medical care costs and have declined as a percentage of overall health care expenditures. Nevertheless, the amount spent on dental care more than doubled between 1970 and 1977. This was not the result of increases in dentists' fees but the product of increases in utilization. Dentists are treating more people, providing more services to each patient, and providing more expensive services (Bailit *et al.* 1979). In fact, the increased intensity of care accounts for about half of the growth in dental care expenditures (Bailit 1986). This is, in part, an outcome of the proliferation of dental insurance plans. When the cost of dental care is wholly or partially removed there is little incentive for the patient to opt for low cost care. This means that the dentist determines what services are needed and, because patients are less likely to reject treatment proposals, the dentist has a major influence on demand for dental care. The Rand Health Insurance Study confirmed that under free care a more expensive mix of services was provided to patients.

Attempts to contain the costs of dental care have involved limiting utilization, changes in the traditional fee-for-service mode of paying the dentist, or the emergence of new forms of payment mechanism. Because some of the emerging forms transfer the economic risk of providing services to the dentist, they have not been welcomed by the profession.

Limiting utilization

Perhaps the easiest strategy for containing dental health care costs is by increasing cost sharing. This not only transfers a greater proportion of expenditure from employers and governments to patients, it constrains costs by reducing the demand for dental care. Increasing co-insurance rates and deductibles, or levying patient fees, reduce both use and expenditures. This reduction in utilization occurs to a greater extent among lower-income groups and, according to current evidence, leads to poorer oral health (Manning *et al.* 1986). An alternative strategy is to reduce the coverage of high cost services which are used by a minority of patients and give priority to basic, more cost-effective services. For example, only 10 per cent of an insured population may receive bridges or crowns but these can account for more than 30 per cent of total costs (Bailit *et al.* 1979).

Reducing system size

A second option for controlling health care costs is to reduce the size of the system. With fewer dentists less care can be provided and dental care expenditures will be lower. In effect, this strategy controls costs by limiting availability and, hence, utilization of services. Apart from the fact that reductions in system size cannot be achieved quickly, nor reversed quickly, the main disadvantage of this approach is that it is likely to reduce use of services by those most in need, i.e., the poor, and will more than likely have an adverse impact on levels of oral health.

Pre-treatment review

Pre-treatment review is a feature of nearly all dental care systems. The NHS General Dental Service and many North American insurance companies require dentists to submit treatment plans for certain high cost procedures or all courses of treatment which exceed a given cost. The aim is to make sure that these treatments are necessary, appropriate, and cost effective. While these systems have the advantage of reducing over-use of some procedures they are inevitably limited in scope. Other mechanisms, such as the analysis of treatment profiles to identify dentists who are over-providing, are also employed in order to limit costs. Nevertheless, deliberate or inadvertent over-prescribing is very difficult to detect.

Capitation payment methods

The methods described above do not challenge the basic fee-for-service mechanism by means of which dentists have usually been paid. Capitation payment methods constitute a major change in this traditional system and shift part of the financial risk in pre-paying dental care to the dentist. Essentially, a dentist enters into a legally enforceable contract to provide a range of dental services as appropriate to a group of subscribing members and is paid a fixed per capita rate for these services. The dentist is paid this fee whether or not subscribing members seek dental care. In a sense, the total fees collected set an upper limit on the cost of care provided to the group as a whole.

Capitation systems emerged because of the supposed disadvantages of paying for health care on a fee-for-service basis. Under fee-for-service methods of reimbursement the dentist has a vested interest in disease, there is a neglect of prevention, and a bias towards over-treatment. Under capitation payment the incentive is for the dentist to prevent disease and to minimize levels or costs of treatments provided. The dentist assumes a financial risk in that treatments provided over and above the capitation fee involve an economic loss. This loss may or may not be compensated by the capitation payments of persons who do not use services in the treatment year. At the time of entering into a contract, the dentist does not know, and may find it difficult to predict, both the levels of treatment required by participants and their utilization behaviour. If both are low the dentist will benefit financially, but if both are high then overall costs may exceed revenues.

Some have argued that capitation leads the dentist to under-treat, to offer lower quality care, and to discourage use of services in order to make a profit from capitation fees. The arguments against this are the ethical standards of the profession and the fact that dentists entering into capitation contracts may be subject to quality control through post-treatment review. In this case, dentists are more likely to alter the mix of services provided to emphasize prevention and early achievement of maintenance care levels in order to minimize future restorative, prosthetic, and surgical treatment needs.

Evidence of the impact of capitation systems on utilization, treatment profiles, and quality of care is limited and not always the product of methodologically sound studies. However, some have compared fee-for-service systems and capitation payment systems and these suggest that capitation is characterized by more prevention and less expensive restorative and prosthodontic procedures. For example, Knowles *et al.* (1987) compared services delivered under fee-for-service and capitation systems and found no differences in utilization rates between the two. However, the mean number of services provided per year was 55 per cent higher and the mean cost per procedure 40 per cent higher among fee-for-service than capitation patients, with the former receiving relatively more restorative work, fixed prosthodontic services, and oral surgery. More diagnostic, preventive, and palliative services were delivered under the capitation system. While this study is better than most, it was not a randomized controlled trial. Consequently, patients' oral health status and treatment needs at entry to the plan were not known and may not have been equivalent. Clearly, the exact impact of capitation on treatment mix and costs remains somewhat uncertain and needs to be assessed using experimental studies. A clinical trial of a capitation scheme for the dental care of children is currently under way in the UK (Coventry *et al.* 1986).

Capitation schemes are most highly developed in the US and are becoming a feature of dental care in Canada, where they are vigorously opposed by the dental profession. Irrespective of their effects on the economics of dental practice, they are believed by some to herald 'the commercialization of dentistry' and 'threaten to compromise the unfettered and independent judgement of the professional' (House 1987). These schemes force economics into clinical decision making and may lead the dentist to provide treament other than that of choice. For this reason, many dental associations believe these schemes place dentists in a dubious ethical position and involve contractual complexities which are destructive for both patient and professional.

Alternative delivery systems

Capitation constitutes a new mode of paying the dentist for providing dental health care to patients (although doctors in Britain's NHS have largely been reimbursed by this method). As such it does not represent an alternative delivery system to traditional fee-for-service practice. While some capitation schemes are often available through Health Maintenance Organizations (HMOs) they are not restricted to HMOs and can be provided through private practice. It is not uncommon, for example, for a practice to consist of a mix of fee-for-service and capitation patients. This may become a feature of the General Dental Service in the UK if capitation is adopted as the mode of payment for the dental care of children. Similarly, group practice does not constitute an alternative delivery system if it consists of two or more fee-for-service practitioners sharing facilities and staff in order to reduce practice overheads.

Other developments in the delivery of dental health care come close to being alternative systems since they involve changes in dental practice organization and payment mechanisms. Some of these have emerged as a result of the desire to contain dental care costs, while some are the product of entrepreneurial activities on the part of dentists and non-dentists. Only a few are strictly new forms of practice organization since there are historical precedents for many. Most are viewed with some suspicion by the organized profession since they are believed to compromise professional integrity and patients' interests. It is also the case that in attempting to preserve professional integrity and maintain the quality of care, the dental profession is protecting its own economic interests in the face of actual and potential competition.

Health maintenance organizations

Health maintenance organizations emerged in the US during the 1970s and became an important component of the attempt to control health care costs. They are legally recognized entities which provide a range of health services under a prepaid capitation system of financing. Where health care is provided as a fringe benefit of employment, employers may offer a contract with an HMO rather than a pre-paid insurance plan. Some HMOs offer dental services, but many do not and contract with groups of dentists for the provision of dental care to enrollees. The dental equivalent of this form of provision is often termed a 'prepaid group practice'.

Closed panel practices

In a closed panel practice an employer or union contracts with a limited number of dentists to provide treatment to employees or members either under prepayment financing or on a salaried basis. These panels are closed in the sense that patients eligible for dental services can only receive treatment at designated facilities from specified dentists. Consequently, the patient does not have free choice of dentist and the dentist must treat all patients eligible under the contract.

Retail dentistry

While retail dentistry does not necessarily imply any change in practice organization or mode of reimbursement, it is novel to the extent that it quite explicitly introduces a business orientation into the provision of dental care. Retail dentistry usually refers to a dental practice, often located in a department store or shopping mall, offering dental services to the general public. These practices use high visibility, convenience of location and extensive advertising to attract a large patient pool. In addition, they may remain open for extended hours and indulge in competitive pricing. Because of their ability to attract patients, they are regarded as a threat to the long-term economic health of traditional dental practice. Such aggressive marketing of dental services is only feasible where dentists are no longer prevented from advertising their services. However, many similar practices are developing in countries such as Canada, where advertising still constitutes a breach of the regulations governing professional conduct. Here patients are attracted by the convenience and location of the service. Those dentists who operate such facilities claim that their patient pool is drawn from that section of the population who do not ordinarily seek dental care because of difficulties in access or other similar barriers.

Competition in dentistry

The development of forms of dental practice competitive in terms of cost and accessibility is inevitable in an era in which health care is coming to be regarded as an industry which exists for the generation of profit rather than as a service to the community. Although the likely impact of these new and emerging forms of dental practice is difficult to determine at the present time, some may well compare favourably with traditional forms of dental care delivery and may alter the existing dental care system considerably.

Certainly, a number of social forces, including deregulation and court decisions concerning advertising, have created tension within the US dental profession and dental care delivery system, leading to change and innovation. The most immediate impact of these forces has been the growth of competition in dentistry (Wotman and Goldman 1982). Dentistry has been actively pushed into the market place at a time when that market is changing if not contracting. Bailit (1982) believes that traditional practices will be able to compete effectively within these market conditions and will not be overtaken by new forms of delivery. Whether traditional or alternative delivery systems come to dominate dental care provision, there seems to be a consensus that competition will lead to forms of practice better able to control costs, improve accessibility, and offer high quality care. While current members of the profession may not be too enthusiastic about the changes occurring within dentistry, some have argued that the oral health of the population will be a major beneficiary, so competition should be accepted and encouraged.

15

Critical appraisals of the health care system

By the middle of the twentieth century, health care systems had become major institutions within the advanced industrialized nations. The scientific discoveries and therapeutic successes of modern medicine, which began in the 1930s and accelerated rapidly during the following decades, were accompanied by an expansion in investment in health care facilities and a massive increase in the numbers of professionals and allied occupations responsible for the delivery of health care. Government policy at this time was largely concerned with improving access to health services. In Britain, 1948 saw the founding of the National Health Service, while in the US the 1960s and 1970s saw the development of federally-funded programmes such as Medicare and Medicaid and the use of indirect tax subsidies to promote the development of private sector health insurance. Federal intervention in Canada's health care system began in 1948 with the National Health Grants Program, which provided funds for the development of the hospital sector. During the 1960s and 1970s, financial inducements were used to encourage the provinces to establish universal insurance schemes whereby all necessary hospital and medical care became available to all residents of Canada irrespective of their financial circumstances.

The belief underlying these major policy initiatives was that better access to health care inevitably led to better health. Britain's NHS was meant to be 'a comprehensive health service designed to secure improvement in the physical and mental health of the people of England and Wales by prevention, diagnosis and treatment of illness' (Ministry of Health 1946). At that time, it was anticipated that health care costs would rise initially, but then fall as the population became healthier and less in need of medical care. This did not happen: the post-war period has been one in which health care costs have risen dramatically both in absolute terms and, in many countries, as a proportion of GNP. In the US, national health expenditures were 5.3 per cent of GNP in 1960 and 10.5 per cent of GNP in 1985. The reasons for this have been touched upon in previous chapters.

The somewhat naive belief in the power of medical science which characterised the immediate post-Second World War period has been tempered by a growing skepticism and an awareness that increased spending on health care has had a limited impact on the health of the population. Evidence which documents the gap between 'inputs' in the form of resources and 'outputs' in the form of health have been the focus of a number of critical appraisals of the health care system. These have been based on a wide range of political philosophies and, as a result, have differed radically in terms of their diagnosis of the problem and preferred solutions.

The input – output problem

The input – output problem can be readily illustrated by examining the performance of Britain's NHS since its inception in the late 1940s to the early 1970s. During this time, expenditures rose by 60 per cent, hospital medical and nursing staff more than doubled and the number of prescriptions issued rose by 40 per cent. Given this increase in resources allocated to health care, a major pay-off in terms of improvements in health was expected. In fact, the benefits have been rather small. Between 1948 and 1970, life expectancy for newborn males rose by 2.4 years, for males aged 25 by 0.8 years, and for males aged 45 by only 0.2 years.

In the US, the massive increase in resources devoted to health care has also failed to bring about major improvements in life expectancy. Between 1900 and 1950, life expectancy at birth for both sexes and all races increased by 21 years. Between 1960 and 1985, a period of scientific advances and an increase in health care expenditure from 27 to 420 billion dollars, the gain in life expectancy was a meagre five years. During the 1980s these gains slowed considerably and appear to have stopped (National Centre for Health Statistics 1987).

Mortality data provide only a limited picture of the population's health and the output of the health care system. They do not take account of the relief of suffering nor of the improvements in the quality of life brought about by medical intervention. Some would argue that these constitute the primary contribution of modern medicine, so that it is misguided to judge the performance of the health care system in terms of its impact on mortality rates. Accordingly, Cochrane (1972) and Powles (1973) have attempted to estimate the changes in morbidity that can be credited to health care. This is not as simple as it might appear, since morbidity data are not routinely collected, are generally unreliable, or do not span the historical period in question. The only data that were available for their analyses were certified spells of sickness absence for employed men. Unfortunately, days of work loss do not provide an accurate measure of morbidity. The data reflect illness behaviour, doctors' ways of managing illness, and work satisfaction, as well as illness. Nevertheless, sickness absence rates worsened rather than improved over the period in question. This picture is also supported by comparing cross-sectional health surveys undertaken in the 1940s (for example, Pearse and Crocker 1949) and 1970s (for example, Wadsworth *et al.* 1971). These studies found high rates of self-reported illness which have not declined over time.

The input–output problem with respect to dentistry is, perhaps, easier to address, if only because reasonably valid and reliable data on oral health are more readily available. Since the 1950s, significant improvements in edentulism rates have been observed and, more recently, there have been dramatic declines in caries rates in children (see Chapter 1).

Cochrane (1972) has argued that assessing the contribution of medical practice in terms of its impact on overall mortality and morbidity rates is both unfair and inconclusive. It is unfair because medicine cannot be blamed for failing to reduce the incidence of, or deaths from, diseases that we do not know how to prevent or cure. The chronic degenerative disorders that are characteristic of late twentieth-century populations are much more complex in terms of prevention and cure than the infectious diseases that were rampant during the nineteenth century. It is inconclusive because it is not possible to isolate the impact of medical effort from other causal factors, such as social and environmental change. As noted in Chapter 1, improvements in oral health cannot be wholly ascribed to the efforts of the organized dental profession; social, economic and environmental factors have played an important part. With respect to dental practice, it might be more apt to ask if the contribution of organized dentistry might not have been achieved at lower cost.

The scientific critique

Cochrane's apparent defence of the contribution of the medical endeavour is not really a defence at all. Rather, he suggests that approaches to the input–output problem which focus on the health of populations have been misguided. The real issue is whether or not the drugs or procedures used in modern medicine (and by implication in dentistry) are effective. Medical practice can only be criticized if it can be shown to be wasting resources on remedies that have no discernible benefit.

Cochrane argues that many supposed therapies in modern medicine are used because they are traditional or established practices and not because there is any scientific evidence to support their efficacy. He advocates the use of randomized controlled trials to ensure that drugs and procedures do more good than harm and to prevent resources being invested in treatments which are useless, dangerous, or entail the consumption of expensive additional resources such as stays in hospital.

In the early seventies, this type of scientific evaluation was less frequent than it is today. Nevertheless, Cochrane was able to draw on studies which showed no discernible benefit was obtained from procedures in common use. One of the more famous and controversial debates concerned the treatment of heart attack patients in coronary care units. Randomized controlled trials which compared home care with care in these units found that the former were just as effective as the latter in terms of the mortality rates of heart attack victims. Yet in the early seventies, coronary care units absorbed the time of 10 per cent of all hospital nurses in the US (Holland 1971).

Although evaluation of drugs and therapeutic procedures is now relatively routine, Cochrane's critique still stands. Resources continue to be wasted on therapies even after they have been shown to be ineffective in randomized controlled trials. The bill paid by the Government of Ontario in providing free drugs to senior citizens and people on social assistance rose from $15 million in 1972 to $480 million in 1985 and there is no doubt that some of this was spent on drugs that have no therapeutic effect. For example, between $3 and $5 million per year is spent on prescriptions for persantine, a drug which is supposed to prevent strokes and heart attacks, but which studies have shown is ineffective. Part of the reason for the continuing use of these preparations is the economic and political power of the pharmaceutical industry, which is able to resist attempts to have such drugs removed from the list of preparations which doctors are allowed to prescribe.

Similar examples can also be found in dentistry. Dentists continue to recall patients at six-month intervals, undertake topical fluoride treatments in fluoridated areas, undertake prophylaxes prior to topical fluoride treatments, and to fill early caries lesions which may remineralize following a more conservative approach. Some of these procedures are ineffective, others inefficient, and for others there is no scientific evidence to support their use. Some would argue that it is in the dentist's economic interests to over-prescribe in this way, while others would see the problem in terms of the failure of new knowledge to permeate the professional community.

The ecological critique

Although critical of the effectiveness and efficiency of much of what passes for modern medicine, Cochrane maintains a commitment to an approach which sees medical intervention as the route to health. Others have no commitment to this approach and argue that the input–output problem stems from the nature of medical practice and the corresponding distribution of resources within health care. That practice is hospital-centred and based on a mechanical or engineering approach to disease.

Hospital-centred practice refers to a type and not a locale of health care (Davies 1979). It has the following characteristics:

1 a curative rather than a preventive orientation,

2 an individualistic rather than an environmental or population approach,

3 an emphasis on high technology,

4 a focus on acute rather than chronic illness, and

5 specialized fragmented treatment rather than holistic care.

The biases inherent in this approach are evident in the

distribution of resources within health care systems. For example, since the inception of the NHS, the hospital sector has claimed the greater part of the total resources allocated to health care. Moreover, over time, it has increased its share of resources, from 56 per cent in 1951 to 66 per cent in 1975, while the proportion spent on general medical and dental services declined during this period. The majority of the increase in funding allocated to hospitals was spent on acute rather than chronic care services, which were, and continue to be, poorly funded. The hospital bias is also reflected in the increasing concentration of manpower in hospitals, with the numbers of doctors practising in hospitals rising more rapidly than the numbers practising in the community. There has of late been a greater emphasis on providing care in the community, particularly for the elderly and the chronic sick. However, in the case of the mentally ill, this has meant a massive reduction in hospital provision without a comparable shift in resources to the community.

This emphasis on acute hospital services and the relative neglect of community services is the outcome of an approach which stresses cure rather than prevention and care. In turn, this is rooted in what has been called the mechanical or engineering approach to health. This is dominated by the belief that improvements in health will result from an understanding of the structure and the function of the body, the ways in which disease affects it, and the discovery of chemical, surgical, or other methods of intervention to counteract these pathological processes. This view pervades not only the organization of health care but also professional education and the character of the patient–practitioner relationship.

The overwhelming emphasis on cure in modern health care systems has led to a relative neglect of the *ecological* approach to health. Extrapolating from his historical analysis, McKeown (1979) suggested that curative medicine is too limited in scope to bring about further improvements in the health of the population. This is because the major health problems in industrialized societies are complex degenerative disorders for which there is little in the way of an effective cure. However, those diseases responsible for the majority of deaths can be prevented by environmental change or changes in personal behaviour. These factors were responsible for past improvements in health (see Chapter 1) and offer the best opportunity for improvements in health in the future. Accordingly, McKeown advocated a shift in health care resources from curative medicine to the prevention of disease and the care of those with chronic, disabling conditions. In arguing that more attention be paid to prevention, McKeown was without doubt that the most significant and productive approach was to bring about changes in personal behaviours, since he believed these to be more significant than the environment in influencing health.

Prevention and health

It is clear that the late 1970s and 1980s have seen a far greater emphasis placed on the prevention of disease. McKeown's work has been influential in spawning the health promotion movement and a concern with the health effects of lifestyles and unfavourable domestic, work, and community environments. Dentistry can rightly claim to have been at the forefront of this movement with its promotion of fluoridation programmes and oral hygiene behaviours, some of which date back to the period following the Second World War. However, it is not altogether clear that the vigour with which prevention and health promotion programmes are advocated by governments is always accompanied by a major shift in health care resources. Some have argued that prevention based on changes in individual behaviour provide governments with the welcome opportunity to abdicate responsibility for the health of their respective populations.

The shift in health care policy which occurred during the late 1970s, and the subsequent emergence of prevention as a key government strategy, were brought about by a concern with the rising costs of health care and continuing high mortality rates from cancer and heart disease. In the analyses contained in official policy documents, governments identified the causes of both these major health problems and allocated responsibility with respect to their solution. Simply put, responsibility for the nation's health was shifted from governments and the health care professions to the individual. This issue of personal responsibility, and the corresponding legitimate role of governments, is most clearly expressed in a publication released by the British government in 1976 with the title *Prevention and Health: Everybody's Business*:

> Much ill-health in Britain today arises from over-indulgence and unwise behaviour. The greatest potential and the greatest problems for preventive medicine now lie in changing behaviour and attitudes to health. The individual can do

much to help himself, his family and the community by accepting more direct responsibility for his own health and well-being.

> The primary responsibility for his own health falls on the individual; the role of the health profession and of the government is limited to ensuring that the public have access to such knowledge as is available about the importance of personal habits to health and, at the very least, no obstacles are placed in the way of those who decide to act on that knowledge. (Department of Health and Social Security 1976)

These crude statements do not embody a radical re-orientation of health care policy. On the contrary, they are little more than a reiteration of traditional approaches to the prevention of disease and ignore the many benefits to be obtained from changes in the environment. That this traditional approach lacks a sophisticated understanding of the origins of ill health is apparent when these statements are reduced to their underlying premises: ill-health is the product of human behaviour and human behaviour can be changed by the provision of information.

The consequence of this view of prevention is an emphasis on health education. One criticism of such an emphasis was addressed in Chapter 11: the provision of information to an individual does not, in and of itself, result in human behaviours conducive to health. However, other more fundamental criticisms have been directed at this traditional approach. Naidoo (1986), for example, has criticized the philosophy of individualism which provides the basis for conventional health education strategies. This philosophy is quite clearly expressed in the statements reproduced above. This philosophy views health as a matter of individual responsibility and free choice. It assumes, quite wrongly, that many of the behaviours damaging to health are freely chosen and can be easily abandoned if only the individual is advised of their untoward effects. Providing such information is the responsibility of governments and professionals, but the responsibility for change lies with the individual. Within the framework of a philosophy which values freedom of choice, education rather than coercion by legal or fiscal means is the strategy by which prevention of illness is to be realized.

Education seeks only to improve levels of knowledge about risks to health and is judged to be successful if this is achieved irrespective of its ultimate impact on behaviour. The main point raised by critics of individualism is not that individual responsibility plays no part in maintaining and improving health, the claim is that approaches which stress individual responsibility and thereby exclude other forces which affect health are going to be limited in their overall impact.

One negative consequence of a stress on individual responsibility for health is its ready translation into 'victim blaming' and the attribution of guilt (Allison 1982). That is, those who succumb to the 'lifestyle diseases' or the 'diseases of choice' are to be condemned as the agents of their own demise. This has recently emerged in the concern expressed for the 'innocent' victims of AIDS: babies born to infected mothers and haemophiliacs who acquired the virus through blood transfusions. This division into the innocent and, by implication, the guilty is not only wholly unwarranted but counterproductive to efforts to contain the disease. It represents nothing more than the confusion of moral judgements and matters of science. Paradoxically, the outcome of such judgements is a call for coercive measures against 'degenerates' who carry and spread the disease. Victim blaming also arises with respect to health issues which are less emotive than AIDS. Allison (1982) refers to a series of television advertisements sponsored by the Workman's Compensation Board and the Construction Safety Association of Ontario which were part of a campaign to reduce work-related accidents. The advertisements depict workers involved in a variety of 'at-risk' behaviours in various industrial settings. No attention is directed towards industrial practices which place these workers at risk or the role of the industry in prevention.

The individualist approach to prevention is limited in that it fails to acknowledge the extent to which health is linked to social and economic conditions which are not within the control of the individual. The individual is relatively powerless to act against a health-damaging environment produced by a society which values profit and economic expansion over and above health. McKinlay (1974) addresses the role of this environment in his analysis of the political economy of illness. There are two aspects to such an analysis. The first concerns the relationship between ill-health and poverty, and the maldistribution of resources within society. The Black Report, for example, identified material deprivation as the cause of social inequalities in health. The second concerns the activities of those industries McKinlay refers to as the 'manufacturers of illness'.

According to McKinlay, the efforts of the health care system can be called 'downstream' activities, devoted as they are to the rescue of the sick. However, this short-term, problem-specific endeavour cannot improve overall levels of health when various interest groups and large-scale profit-oriented corporations are operating 'up-stream' and constantly adding to the pool of those in need of rescue. Problems such as lung cancer, heart disease, obesity, alcoholism, and road traffic accidents are linked to organizations such as the tobacco and food industries who spend billions of dollars a year promoting the various at-risk behaviours health educators are trying to change. The battle is an unequal one. The tobacco industry commands massive resources and has access to more sophisticated persuasive techniques than those who seek to counter their efforts. McKinlay believes that these persuasive techniques are effective because they successfully tie at-risk behaviours to dominant cultural values and images. In this regard it is futile to talk of free choice when considering these behaviours. Such choices are shaped and limited by environmental factors and commercial interests which profit from unhealthy lifestyles. Because free choice is unrealistic, McKinlay advocates legislative action to curb the activities of the manufacturers of illness.

McKinlay's approach to health is often called a 'structuralist' approach. This seeks to improve health by means of interventions designed to change the social, economic, and physical environment in which we live. Such changes only come about as a result of political action by communities and governments, so that health cannot be deemed to be solely an individual responsibility.

Individualist and structuralist strategies compared

A good illustration of the differences between individualist and structuralist perspectives on health is to be found in a recent analysis of strategies for enhancing the nutritional status of children (Love and Kalnins 1984). Largely as a result of the increased consumption of processed and refined foods, children have higher intakes of saturated animal fats and sugars, and lower intakes of dairy products, whole grain cereals, and fresh fruit and vegetables than is desirable. In children, high fat and high sugar diets have been linked to a number of health problems, including dental decay.

From the individualist perspective these health problems are seen to be the product of unhealthy aspects of lifestyle and the solution seen to reside in education to raise levels of knowledge of nutritional issues and to change attitudes and behaviour. As a consequence, health educators base their efforts on a body of research which focuses on children's nutritional knowledge, attitudes, and behaviours; the influence of the family on the development of these psychological variables; and children's own concepts of health and ways of staying well.

Surveys of knowledge, attitudes, and behaviours provide a baseline against which to judge the effect of health education programmes, to identify specific areas where improvement is required, and, by exploring the links between behaviour and psychological variables, to develop the most appropriate strategy for bringing about behaviour change. Research on the family is based on the assumption that mothers are important educators with respect to children and that their knowledge, attitudes, and behaviour are transmitted to the child both formally and informally, and are carried into adulthood. This provides the rationale for interventions at the level of the family and efforts to improve the nutritional knowledge and practices of mothers. Studies have found little evidence to support the existence of this effect. Finally, research on children's concepts of health helps health educators to couch health education messages which are appropriate for the level of cognitive development of their target audience.

The structuralist approach largely ignores the individual and the family, but focuses instead on broader social and political changes without which the nutritional status of children will not be improved. Poverty, the food industry, and television advertising are the major targets for change, since all are believed to have a major influence on the quality of the diet.

Although the industrialized nations are affluent, substantial numbers of people live at or below the poverty line. Most vulnerable are the elderly living alone, families with four or more children, and single parent families. Those on low incomes spend less on food than the more affluent and because of local market conditions often pay higher prices for food of an inferior quality. As a consequence, the consumption of fruit and vegetables decreases and the consumption of starchy foods increases with declining income. These differences in access to a nutritious diet are a political problem that cannot be solved by individual behaviour change. A second constraint on the quality of diets is the quality of food that is available. The increase in corporate control over the whole process of food production, from agriculture to food processing and retailing, has, according to some researchers, been associated with a decline in the nutritional value of foods and a decline in competition between producers. The activities of the food industry are supported by television advertising, much of which is directed at children. Currently, about 60 per cent of such advertising is for edible products: typically, confectionery, snacks and soft drinks which are high in sugar, or fast foods which are high in saturated fats. Studies have shown that television advertising does have an influence on children's preferences and requests for foods, particularly highly sugared snacks. Rather than attempting to counter the influence of the food and advertising industries by education, structuralists believe that controls on their activities are necessary and more effective. The role of health education within this strategy is more concerned with informing consumers of the way in which their dietary choices are shaped by commercial interests and the way these interests can be challenged by political action.

Health promotion

Health promotion is the name given to a more comprehensive strategy aimed at improving the health of the population. It emerged as a result of the seminal work of Lalonde (1974) and has gained momentum following the increasing recognition of the importance of external influences on health and the constraints on behaviour change.

> The terms health promotion and health education are not interchangeable. Health promotion covers all aspects of those activities that seek to improve the health status of individuals and communities. It includes both health education and all attempts to produce environmental and legislative change conducive to good health. (Speller 1985)

In recognizing the role of the individual *and* the environment in determining levels of health, this more comprehensive strategy is a synthesis of the concerns raised by the individualist and structuralist perspectives. Here the individual is not accorded sole responsibility for his or her health, nor is the individual seen as the victim of social forces over which they have no control. Rather, individuals can do much to improve their health, although they are ultimately limited by the social and economic circumstances within which they live. The task of health promotion is to identify all barriers to health, individual and societal, and to find ways to remove these barriers to healthy choices.

Canada has one of the most highly developed health promotion programmes, combining interventions directed at the individual with legislation to reduce threats to health. Programmes such as PARTICIPaction attempt to increase public awareness of positive health practices and encourage individuals to modify at-risk behaviours. At the same time, local by-laws have been passed to prohibit or limit smoking in the workplace and the federal government is currently in the process of instigating legislation to effect a complete ban on the advertising of cigarettes and to prevent tobacco companies from sponsoring sporting and cultural events. This goes far beyond the current state of affairs in most other advanced economies, where tobacco companies are subject only to voluntary restraint.

The case of cigarette advertising illustrates quite clearly the political nature of health issues. The tobacco industry has mounted a major political campaign in Canada and is engaged in extensive lobbying activities in order to neutralize the proposed legislation and to protect its economic interests. The industry expressly denies the connection between smoking and ill-health, in spite of the fact that 35,000 Canadians a year die from smoking-related diseases, and also claims that a ban on advertising is a breach of human rights and freedom of expression. Similarly, the British government recently decided not to introduce legislation banning the use of highly inflammable foams in furniture, in spite of the fact that 300 to 400 people die annually from inhaling toxic gases given off by burning foams. Lobbying by the furniture industry concerned about the economic effects of such a ban were a major factor influencing that decision. The decision was reversed following the intervention of senior fire officers and pressure from consumer groups.

Such political struggles are more likely in situations where legislation to protect or promote health challenges major interest groups within a society. The one major exception to this rule has been the controversy over the fluoridation of public water supplies. Fluoridation has been one of the most successful of all public health initiatives. It is effective, reducing decay in children by up to

50 per cent. It is cheap to implement and administer and does not require any cooperation on the part of those who benefit from its effects. Numerous studies have provided convincing evidence that, at optimum levels, it has no harmful effects. Nevertheless, many communities do not have the benefit of fluoridation because of opposition from a variety of local and national groups.

Early opponents of fluoridation were connected with the health food movement, belonged to the Christian Scientist church, or were fringe medical practitioners. Even individuals, opposing fluoridation on the basis of coercion and human rights, have used the courts to block fluoridation schemes. In many communities, such schemes may only be implemented if a majority is obtained in a local referendum. By exploiting society's currently heightened concerns about health and disease, antifluoridationists are able more often than not to influence the outcomes of referenda negatively and defeat fluoridation proposals (Easley 1985). Although their motives are difficult to understand, there is no doubt that the antifluoridationists are a potent political force and need to be challenged by an equally effective political response. Again, this serves to emphasize the extent to which health is a political as well as a personal issue.

Further reading

Comprehensive texts

Aiken, L. and Mechanic, D. (eds) (1986) *Applications of Social Science to Clinical Medicine and Health Policy*, New Brunswick: Rutgers University Press.

Cohen, L. and Bryant, P. (eds) (1984) *Social Sciences and Dentistry: A Critical Bibliography*, Vol. II, London: Fédération Dentaire Internationale/Quintessence.

Steptoe, A. and Mathews, A. (eds) (1984) *Health Care and Human Behaviour*, London: Academic Press.

Psychology and dental practice

Dworkin, S., Ference, T. and Giddon, D. (1978) *Behavioral Science and Dental Practice*, Saint Louis: The C. V. Mosby Co.

Geboy, M. (1985) *Communication and Behaviour Management in Dentistry*, Baltimore: Williams & Wilkins.

Ingersoll, B. (1982) *Behavioral Aspects in Dentistry*, New York: Appleton-Century-Crofts.

Kent, G. (1984) *The Psychology of Dental Care*, Bristol: Wright.

Sociology and medicine

Hart, N. (1985) *The Sociology of Health and Medicine*, Ormskirk: Causeway Press Ltd.

Morgan, M., Calnan, M. and Manning, N. (1985) *Sociological Approaches to Health and Medicine*, Beckenham: Croom Helm.

Patrick, D. and Scambler, G. (1986) *Sociology as Applied to Medicine*, London: Baillière Tindall.

References

Ackerman, C. (1987) *The Emotional and Physiological Responses of Dentists and their Patients during Administration of a Local Anaesthetic*, PhD thesis, York University, unpublished.

Allison, K. (1982) 'Health education; self-responsibility *vs* blaming the victim', *Health Education* 20: 11–13.

Anderson, R. and Newman, J. (1973) 'Societal and individual determinants of medical care utilization in the US', *Millbank Memorial Fund Quarterly* 51: 95–124.

Anderson, R. (1981) 'The changes in the dental health of 12-year-old schoolchildren in two Somerset schools', *British Dental Journal* 150: 218–21.

Anderson, R., Bradnock, G. and James, P. (1981) 'The changes in the dental health of 12-year-old school children in Shropshire', *British Dental Journal* 150: 278–81.

Andrews, F. and Withey, S. (1974) 'Developing measures of perceived quality of life', *Social Indicators Research* 7: 28–37.

Auerbach, S., Kendall, P. and Cuttler, H. (1976) 'Anxiety, locus of control, type of preparatory information and adjustment to dental surgery', *Journal of Consulting and Clinical Psychology* 44: 809–18.

Ayer, W. and Corah, N. (1984) 'Behavioral factors influencing dental treatment', in L. Cohen and P. Bryant (eds) *Social Sciences and Dentistry: A Critical Bibliography*, Vol II, London: FDI/Quintessence.

Ayer, W. and Morretti, R. (1985) 'Stress in dentistry: where's the evidence?', *Journal of the American Dental Association* 110: 22.

Bader, J. (1982) 'Auxiliary turnover in 13 dental offices', *Journal of the American Dental Association* 104: 307–12.

Bailit, H., Raskin, M., Reisine, S. and Chiriboga, D. (1979) 'Controlling the cost of dental care', *American Journal of Public Health* 69: 699–703.

Bailit, H. (1982) 'Traditional and emerging forms of dental practice: another view', *American Journal of Public Health* 72: 662–4.

Bailit, H. (1986) 'Future financing of health care', *Journal of Dental Education* 50: 119–24.

Banks, M., Beresford, S., Morrell, D., Waller, J. and Watkins, C. (1975) 'Factors influencing demand for primary medical care among women aged 20–44 years', *International Journal of Epidemiology* 4: 189–95.

Basker, R., Sturdee, D. and Davenport, J. (1978) 'Patients with burning mouths', *British Dental Journal* 145: 9–16.

Baum, B. (1981) 'Research on aging and oral health: an assessment of current status and future needs', *Special Care in Dentistry* 1: 156–65.

Beal, J. and Dickson, S. (1974) 'Diet and dental health', *Health Education Journal* 33: 8–12.

Beal, J. (1983) 'Social factors and preventive dentistry', in J. Murray (ed.) *The Prevention of Dental Disease*, Oxford: Oxford University Press.

Beck, J. (1984) 'The epidemiology of dental diseases in the elderly', *Gerodontology* 3: 5–15.

Beck, J. and Hunt, R. (1985) 'Oral health status in the US: problems of special patients', *Journal of Dental Education* 49: 407–25.

Beck, J., Kohout, F., Hunt, R. and Heckert, D. (1986) 'Root caries: physical, mental and psychosocial correlates in an elderly population', *Gerodontics* 3: 242–7.

Becker, M. (1977) 'Selected psychological models and correlates of individual health related behaviour', *Medical Care* 15, Supplement: 27–46.

Beecher, H. (1956) 'Relationship of significance of wound to the pain experienced', *American Medical Association Journal* 161: 1609–15.

Bergner, M. and Bobbitt, B. (1981) 'The sickness impact profile: development and final revision of a health status measure', *Medical Care* 19: 787–805.

Berkey, D., Call, R. and Loupe, M. (1985) 'Oral health perceptions and self-esteem in non-institutionalized older adults', *Gerodontics* 1: 213–16.

Berkman, L. and Syme, S. (1979) 'Social networks, host resistance and mortality: a nine-year follow-up study of Almeda County residents', *American Journal of Epidemiology* 109: 186–204.

Birch, S. (1985) 'NHS patient charges and the privatisation of dental care', *British Dental Journal* 159: 377–8.

Blaikie, D. C. (1979) 'Cultural barriers to preventive dentistry', *Australian Dental Journal* 24: 398–401.

Blane, D. (1985) 'An assessment of the Black Report's explanation of health inequalities', *Sociology of Health and Illness* 7: 423–45.

Blane, D. (1986) 'Health professions', in D. Patrick and G. Scambler (eds) *Sociology as Applied to Medicine*, London: Baillière Tindall.

Blaxter, M. (1984) 'Equity and consultation rates in general practice', *British Medical Journal* 6345: 1963–6.

Blinkhorn, A. and Verity, J. (1979) 'Assessment of the readability of dental health education literature', *Community Dentistry and Oral Epidemiology* 7: 195–9.

Blinkhorn, A. (1981) 'Dental health education', in G. Slack, *Dental Public Health*, Bristol: John Wright & Sons.

Borysenko, M., Turesky, S., Borysenko, J., Quimby, F. and Benson, H. (1980) 'Stress and dental caries in the rat', *Journal of Behavioral Medicine* 3: 233–9.

Boulton, M., Tuckett, D., Olson, C. and Williams, A. (1986) 'Social class and the general practice consultation', *Sociology of Health and Illness* 8: 325–50.

Brown, G. and Harris, T. (1979) *The Social Origins of Depression*, London: Tavistock.

Bullen, M. (1982) *The Utilisation of Dental Services by Ontario Adults*, MSc thesis, Faculty of Dentistry, University of Toronto.

Burman, D. (1988) *A Study of Dentists' Response Styles to Negative Patient Affect*, PhD thesis, University of Toronto, in progress.

Burstein, A. and Burstein, M. (1979) 'Injection pain: memory, expectation and experienced pain', *New York Journal of Dentistry* 49: 183–5.

Burt, B. (1978) 'Influences for change in the dental health status of populations: an historical perspective', *Journal of Public Health Dentistry* 38: 272–88.

Burt, B. (1983) 'The epidemiology of oral disease', in D. Striffler, W.

Young and B. Burt (eds) *Dentistry, Dental Practice and the Community*, Philadelphia: W. B. Saunders.

Burt, B. (1985) 'The future of the caries decline', *Journal of Public Health Dentistry* 45: 261–9.

Byrne, P. and Long, B. (1976) *Doctors Talking to Patients*, London: HMSO.

Carmichael, C., Rugg-Gunn, A., French, A. and Cranage, J. (1980) 'The effect of fluoridation upon the relationship between caries experience and social class in 5-year-old children in Newcastle and Northumberland', *British Dental Journal* 149: 163–7.

Carmichael, C., French, A., Rugg-Gunn, A. and Furness, J. (1984) 'The relationship between social class and caries experience in five-year-old children in Newcastle and Northumberland after twelve years of fluoridation', *Community Dental Health* 1: 47–54.

Cartwright, A. (1964) *Human Relations and Hospital Care*, London: Routledge & Kegan Paul.

Cartwright, A. and O'Brien, M. (1976) 'Social class variations in health care', in *The Sociology of the NHS*, Sociological Review (Monograph) 22.

Cartwright, A. and Anderson, R. (1981) *General Practice Revisited: A Second Study of Patients and Their Doctors*, London: Tavistock.

Charette, A. (1986) 'Dental care utilisation in Canada. Analysis of the Canada Health Survey (1978–79)', unpublished, University of Ottawa.

Chauncey, H. (1978) 'The incidence of coronal caries in normal aging male adults', *Journal of Dental Research* 57 (special issue): 148, abstract no. 296.

Chiodo, G., Rosenstein, D. and Clarke, J. (1986) 'Counselling principles for more effective patient education', *Community Dentistry and Oral Epidemiology* 14: 190–2.

Christen, A. (1984) 'Stress and distress in dental practice', in H. Goldman, S. Hartman and J. Messite (eds) *Occupational Hazards in Dentistry*, Chicago: Yearbook Medical Publishers.

Christen, A., Nevin, R. and Christen, J. (1986) 'Active coping strategies: from self-help to psychological counselling', *Dental Clinics of North America* 30: S67–S78.

Claridge, G. (1970) *Drugs and Human Behaviour*, London: Allen Lane.

Clark, G., Beemsterboer, P. and Rugh, J. (1981) 'Nocturnal masseter muscle activity and the symptoms of mandibular dysfunction', *Journal of Oral Rehabilitation* 8: 279–83.

Clark, J. and Phillips, S. (1981) 'Stress and the dental assistant', *Dental Assistant* 50: 31–3.

Cochrane, A. (1972) *Effectiveness and Efficiency: Random Reflections on the Health Service*, London: The Nuffield Provincial Hospitals Trust.

Cohen, L. and Jago, J. (1976) 'Toward the formulation of socio-dental indicators', *International Journal of Health Services* 6: 681–7.

Cohen, L. (1978) 'Implications of findings for dental care across cultures', *International Dental Journal* 28: 283–8.

Collett, H. (1969) 'Influence of dentist–patient relationship on attitudes and adjustment to dental treatment', *Journal of the American Dental Association* 79: 879–84.

Comarroff, J. (1976) 'Communicating information about non-fatal

illness: the strategies of a group of general practitioners', *Sociological Review* 24: 269–90.
Cooper, C., Mallinger, M. and Kahn, R. (1978) 'Identifying sources of occupational stress among dentists', *Journal of Occupational Psychology* 51: 227–34.
Cooper, C., Watts, J. and Kelly, M. (1987) 'Job satisfaction, mental health, and job stressors among general dental practitioners in the UK', *British Dental Journal* 158: 77–81.
Corah, N. (1969) 'Development of a dental anxiety scale', *Journal of Dental Research* 48: 596–602.
Corah, N. (1974) 'The dental practitioner and preventive health behaviour', *Health Education Monographs* 2: 226–35.
Corah, N. (1984) 'Reduction of patient stress and the patient–dentist relationship', *New York State Dental Journal* 50: 478–9.
Corah, N., O'Shea, R. and Bissell, D. (1985) 'The dentist–patient relationship: mutual perceptions and behaviors', *Journal of the American Dental Association* 113: 253–5.
Coventry, P., Holloway, P. and Lennon, A. (1986) 'A capitation system for the treatment of children in the general dental services', *British Dental Journal* 160: 174–7.
Craig, K. and Prkachin, K. (1978) 'Social modelling influences on sensory decision theory and neuropsychological indexes of pain', *Journal of Personality and Social Psychology* 36: 805–15.
Culyer, A. J. (ed.) (1983) *Health Indicators*, Oxford: Martin Robertson.
Curson, I. and Coplans, M. (1970) 'The need for sedation in conservative dentistry', *British Dental Journal* 125: 18–22.
Cushing, A., Sheiham, A. and Maizels, J. (1986) 'Developing socio-dental indicators — the social impact of dental disease', *Community Dental Health* 3: 3–17.
Davies, C. (1979) 'Hospital-centred health care: policies and politics in the NHS', in P. Atkinson and M. Murcott (eds) *Prospects for the National Health*, Beckenham: Croom Helm.
Davis, P. (1976) 'Compliance structures and the delivery of health care: the case of dentistry', *Social Science and Medicine* 10: 329–35.
Davis, P. (1980) *The Social Context of Dentistry*, Beckenham: Croom Helm.
Davis, P. (1981) 'Culture, inequality and the pattern of dental care in New Zealand', *Social Science and Medicine* 15A: 801–5.
Department of Health and Social Security (1976) *Prevention and Health: Everybody's Business*, London: HMSO.
Diesendorf, M. (1986) 'The mystery of declining tooth decay', *Nature* 322: 125–9.
Douglass, C. and Cole, K. (1979) 'Utilization of dental services in the United States', *Journal of Dental Education* 43: 223–38.
Douglass, C., Gillings, D., Sollecito, W. and Gammon, M. (1983) 'National trends in the prevalence and severity of periodontal disease', *Journal of the American Dental Association* 107: 405–12.
Dunlap, E. and Stewart, D. (1982) 'Survey suggests less stress in group offices', *Dental Economics*, February: 46–56.
Dworkin, S., Ference, T. and Giddon, D. (1978) *Behavioral Science and Dental Practice*, St Louis: C. V. Mosby Co.

Dworkin, S. and Chen, A. (1982) 'Pain in clinical and laboratory contexts', *Journal of Dental Research* 61: 772–4.

Easley, M. (1985) 'The new antifluoridationists: who are they and how do they operate?', *Journal of Public Health Dentistry* 45: 133–41.

Eccles, J. and Powell, M. (1967) 'The health of dentists: a survey in South Wales, 1965/6', *British Dental Journal* 123: 379–83.

Egbert, L., Battit, G., Welch, C. and Bartlett, M. (1964) 'Reduction of post-operative pain by encouragement and instruction of patients', *New England Journal of Medicine* 270: 825–7.

Enbom, L., Magnusson, T. and Wall, G. (1986) 'Occlusal wear in miners', *Swedish Dental Journal* 10: 165–70.

Epsom, J. (1969) 'The mobile health clinic: a report on the first year's work', in D. Tuckett and J. Kaufert (eds) (1978) *Basic Readings in Medical Sociology*, London: Tavistock.

Epstein, S. (1987) 'Importance of psychosocial and behavioral factors in food ingestion in the elderly and their ramifications on oral health', *Gerodontics* 3: 23–5.

Ettinger, R. and Beck, J. (1982) 'The new elderly: what can the dental profession expect?', *Geriatric Dentistry* 2: 62–9.

Ettinger, R. and Beck, J. (1983) 'Medical and psychosocial risk factors in the dental treatment of the elderly', *International Dental Journal* 33: 292–300.

Ettinger, R. (1987) 'Oral disease and its effect on the quality of life', *Gerodontics* 3: 103–6.

Fassler, D. (1980) 'Reducing preoperative anxiety in children', *Patient Counseling and Health Education* 2: 130–4.

Field, D. (1976) 'The social definition of health', in D. Tuckett (ed.) *An Introduction to Medical Sociology*, London: Tavistock.

Fitzpatrick, R., Hopkins, A. and Harvard-Watts, O. (1983) 'Social dimensions of healing', *Social Science and Medicine* 17: 501–10.

Fitzpatrick, R. (1986a) 'Society and changing patterns of disease', in D. Patrick and G. Scambler (eds) *Sociology as Applied to Medicine*, London: Baillière Tindall.

Fitzpatrick, R. (1986b) 'Social causes of disease', in D. Patrick and G. Scambler (eds) *Sociology as Applied to Medicine*, London: Baillière Tindall.

Fleck-Kandath, C., Tedesco, L., Keffer, M., Christersson, L., Grossi, S., Genco, R. and Albino, A. (1988) 'Distress and oral health behaviour reports', *Journal of Dental Research* 67 (special issue): abstract no. 1322.

Forgione, A. and Clarke, R. (1974) 'Comments on an empirical study of the causes of dental fears', *Journal of Dental Research* 53: 496–501.

Forrest, W. (1978) 'Stresses and self-destructive behaviors of dentists', *Dental Clinics of North America* 22: 361–71.

Forster, D. (1976) 'Social class differences in sickness and general practitioner consultations', *Health Trends* 8: 29–32.

Frazier, J., Jenny, J., Bagramian, R., Robinson, E. and Proshek, J. (1977) 'Provider expectations and consumer perceptions of the importance and value of dental care', *American Journal of Public Health* 67: 37–43.

Frazier, J. (1978) 'A new look at dental health education in community programmes', *Dental Hygiene* 52: 176–86.

Freidson, E. (1970) *Profession of Medicine*, New York: Dodd, Mead & Co.

Freidson, E. (1986) 'The medical profession in transition', in L. Aiken and D. Mechanic (eds) *Applications of Social Science to Clinical Medicine and Health Policy*, New Brunswick: Rutgers University Press.

Friedman, M. and Rosenman, R. (1974) *Type A Behavior and Your Heart*, New York: Knopf.

Gale, E. and Ayer, W. (1969) 'Treatment of dental phobias', *Journal of the American Dental Association* 73: 1304–7.

Gale, E. (1972) 'Fears of the dental situation', *Journal of Dental Research* 15: 964–6.

Gale, E., Carlsson, S., Erikson, A. and Jontell, M. (1984) 'Effects of dentists' behavior on patients' attitudes', *Journal of the American Dental Association* 109: 444–6.

Geboy, M. and Muzzio, T. (1985) 'The geriatric patient', in M. Geboy (ed.) *Communication and Behavior Management in Dentistry*, Baltimore: Williams & Wilkins.

George, J., Block, M., Milone, C. and Hollister, W. (1986) *Stress Management for the Dental Team*, Philadelphia: Lea & Febiger.

Gerstl, E. (1959) *Career Commitments and Style of Life in Three Middle-Class Occupations*, PhD thesis, University of Minnesota, unpublished.

Gift, H. (1984) 'The utilization of professional dental services', in L. Cohen and P. Bryant (eds) *Social Science and Dentistry: A Critical Bibliography*, Vol II, London: FDI/Quintessence.

Glass, R. (1966) *Mortality of New England Dentists, 1921–60*, US Department of Health Education and Welfare, Washington.

Goode, W. (1960) 'Encroachment, charlatanism and the emerging profession: psychiatry, sociology and medicine', *American Sociological Review* 25: 902–14.

Goodwin, W., Starks, D., Green, T. and Koran, A. (1981) 'Identification of sources of stress in practice by recent dental graduates', *Journal of Dental Education* 45: 220–1.

Gove, W. (1979) 'The relationship between sex, marital status and mortality', *American Journal of Sociology* 79: 45–67.

Graves, R. and Stamm, J. (1985) 'Oral health status in the United States: prevalence of dental caries', *Journal of Dental Education* 49: 341–51.

Graves, R., Bohannan, H., Disney, J., Stamm, J. and Bader, J. (1986) 'Recent dental caries and treatment patterns in US children', *Journal of Public Health Dentistry* 46: 23–9.

Gray, P., Todd, J., Slack, G. and Bulman, J. (1970) *Adult Dental Health in England and Wales in 1968*, London: HMSO.

Green, L. (1979) 'National policy in the promotion of health', *International Journal of Health Education* 22: 161–70.

Green, R. and Green, A. (1985) 'Adult attitudes towards dentistry among dental attenders in South Wales', *British Dental Journal* 161: 157–60.

Gupta, O. (1966) 'Psychosomatic factors in periodontal disease', *Dental Clinics of North America*, March 11–21.

Hand, J., Hunt, R. and Beck, J. (1988) 'Incidence of coronal and root caries in an older adult population', *Journal of Public Health Dentistry* 48: 14–19.

Hannay, D. (1980) 'The iceberg of illness and trivial consultations', *Journal of the Royal College of General Practitioners* 30: 551–4.

Hardwick, J. (1960) 'The incidence and distribution of caries throughout the ages in relation to the Englishman's diet', *British Dental Journal* 108: 9–17.

Hart, N. (1985) *The Sociology of Health and Medicine*, Ormskirk: Causeway Press.

Haug, M. (1975) 'The deprofessionalization of everyone?', *Sociological Focus* 8: 197–213.

Hausen, H., Heinonen, O. and Paunio, I. (1981) 'Caries in permanent dentition and social class of children participating in public dental care in fluoridated and non-fluoridated areas', *Community Dentistry and Oral Epidemiology* 9: 289–91.

Haynes, S. and Feinleb, M. (1980) 'Women, work and coronary heart disease: prospective findings from the Framingham heart study', *American Journal of Public Health* 770: 133–41.

Helkimo, M. (1974) 'Studies on the function and dysfunction of the masticatory system', *Swedish Dental Journal* 67: 165–82.

Helman, C. (1984) *Culture, Health and Illness*, Bristol: John Wright & Sons Ltd.

Hendrix, W. (1986) 'Dental stress model and assessment questionnaire', *Dental Clinics of North America* 30: S1–S11.

Hirschman, R. (1980) 'Physiological feedback and stress reduction', in B. Ingersoll (ed.) *Behavioral Approaches to Pain, Fear and Stress*, Symposium of the Society of Behavioral Medicine, New York.

Holland, W. (1971) 'Clinicians and the use of medical resources', *The Hospital* 67 (London): 236–9.

Hollander, F. and Dunning, J. (1939) 'A study by age and sex of the incidence of dental caries in over 12,000 persons', *Journal of Dental Research* 18: 43–60.

Horowitz, H. (1985) 'The National Institute of Dental Research's 1985 Survey of Working and Senior Adults', *Journal of Public Health Dentistry* 4: 227–8.

House, R. C. (1987) 'The patient and profession at risk: alternative delivery systems', *Journal of the Canadian Dental Association* 6: 447–53.

Howard, J., Cunningham, D., Rechnitzer, P. and Goode, R. (1976) 'Stress in the job and career of a dentist', *Journal of the American Dental Association* 93: 630–6.

Hunt, R. (1985) 'Edentulism and oral health problems among elderly rural Iowans', *American Journal of Public Health* 75: 1177–81.

Hunt, S. and McEwen, J. (1980) 'The development of a subjective health indicator', *Sociology of Health and Illness* 2: 231–45.

Hunt, S., McEwen, J. and McKenna, S. P. (1986) *Measuring Health Status*, Beckenham: Croom Helm.

Illsley, R. (1980) *Professional or Public Health?* London: Nuffield Provincial Hospitals Trust.

Infante, P. and Owen, G. (1975) 'Dental caries and levels of treatment for schoolchildren by geographical region, socioeconomic status, race and size of community', *Journal of Public Health Dentistry* 35: 19–27.

Ingersoll, B. (1982) *Behavioral Aspects in Dentistry*, New York: Appleton-Century-Crofts.

Iwata, B. and Beckford, C. (1981) 'Behavioral research in preventive dentistry: educational and contingency management approaches to the problem of patient compliance', *Journal of Applied Behavior Analysis* 14: 111–20.

Jackson, D. (1987) 'Has the decline of dental caries in English children made water fluoridation both unnecessary and uneconomic?', *British Dental Journal* 162: 170–3.

Jackson, E. (1974) 'Managing dental fears: a tentative code of practice', *Journal of Oral Medicine* 29: 96–101.

Jackson, E. (1978) 'Patients' perceptions of dentistry', in P. Weinstein (ed.) *Advances in Behavioral Research in Dentistry*, Seattle: University of Washington.

Jenkins, P., Feldman, B. and Stirrups, D. (1984) 'The effect of social class and dental features on referrals for orthodontic advice and treatment', *British Dental Journal* 158: 24–6.

Jenny, J. and Proshek, J. (1986) 'Visibility and prestige of occupations and the importance of dental appearance', *Journal of the Canadian Dental Association* 52: 987–9.

Jepson, C. (1986) 'Some behavioural aspects of dental–patient compliance', *Journal of Dental Practice Administration* 3: 117–22.

Johnson, R. and Baldwin, C. (1968) 'Relationship of maternal anxiety to the behaviour of young children undergoing dental extraction', *Journal of Dental Research* 47: 801–5.

Johnson, T. (1972) *Professions and Power*, London: Macmillan.

Johnston, D., Grainger, R. and Ryan, R. (1986) 'The decline of dental caries in Ontario schoolchildren', *Journal of the Canadian Dental Association* 52: 411–17.

Kasl, S. and Cobb, S. (1966) 'Health behaviour, illness behaviour and sick role behaviour', *Archives of Environmental Health* 12: 246–66.

Kay, E. and Blinkhorn, A. (1987) 'Some factors related to dentists' decisions to extract teeth', *Community Dental Health* 4: 3–10.

Kegeles, S., Lund, K. and Weisenberg, M. (1978) 'Acceptance by children of a daily home mouthrinse programme', *Social Science and Medicine* 12: 199–210.

Kent, G. (1984) *The Psychology of Dental Care*, Bristol: John Wright & Sons.

Kincey, J., Bradshaw, P. and Ley, P. (1975) 'Patients' satisfaction and reported acceptance of advice in general practice', *Journal of the Royal College of General Practitioners* 25: 558–62.

Kitamura, M. and Kiyak, A. (1986) 'Predictors of root caries in the elderly', *Community Dentistry and Oral Epidemiology* 14: 34–8.

Kiyak, A. (1984) 'Utilization of dental services by the elderly', *Gerodontology* 3: 17–25.

Kleinknecht, R., Klepac, R. and Alexander, L. (1973) 'Origins and characteristics of fear of dentistry', *Journal of the American Dental Association* 86: 482–8.

Kleinknecht, R. and Bernstein, D. (1978) 'The assessment of dental fear', *Behavioural Therapy* 9: 626–34.

Kleinknecht, R. (1978) 'Fear of dentistry: its development, measurement and implications', in P. Weinstein (ed.) *Advances in Behavioral Research in Dentistry*, Seattle: University of Washington.

Klepac, R. (1975) 'Successful treatment of avoidance of dentistry by desensitisation or by increasing pain tolerance', *Journal of Behavior Therapy and Experimental Psychiatry* 6: 307–10.

Klima, R. and McIver, J. (1979) 'Body image, self-concept and the orthodontic patient', *American Journal of Orthodontics*, 75: 507–17.

Knowles, M., Hutgler, M. and Schacter, M. (1987) 'A balance of containment incentives: comparison of capitation and fee for service payment systems', *American Public Health Association*, abstract no. 2013.

Kobasa, S. (1979) 'Stressful life events, personality and health: an inquiry into hardiness', *Journal of Personality and Social Psychology* 37: 1–11.

Korsch, B., Gozzi, E. and Francis, V. (1969) 'Gaps in doctor–patient communication: patients' response to medical advice', *New England Journal of Medicine* 280: 535–40.

Koshi, E. (1971) 'Health status of adolescent school girls in a region of Alambagh, Lucknow', *Indian Journal of Medical Science* 25: 376–83.

Krasner, D. (1978) 'Stress as a distal etiological factor in dental disease', *Journal of Preventive Dentistry* 5: 24–7.

Kydd, J. (1959) 'Psychosomatic aspects of temporomandibular joint dysfunction', *Journal of the American Dental Association* 59: 31–4.

Lalonde, M. (1974) *A New Perspective on the Health of Canadians*, Ottawa: Queen's Printer.

Lang, R. (1981) 'Stress in dentistry — it can kill you', *Oral Health* 71: 6–8.

Lang-Runtz, H. (1984) 'Stress in dentistry — it can kill you', *Journal of the Canadian Dental Association* 7: 539–41.

Larson, M. (1978) *The Rise of Professionalism: A Sociological Analysis*, Los Angeles: California University Press.

Last, J. (1963) 'The clinical iceberg: completing the clinical picture in general practice', *The Lancet* 2: 28–31.

Lautch, H. (1971) 'Dental phobia', *British Journal of Psychiatry* 119: 151–8.

Lazarus, R. (1966) *Psychological Stress and the Coping Process*, New York: McGraw-Hill.

Leake, J. (1984) 'Expenditures on dental services in Canada, Canadian Provinces and Territories 1960–80', *Journal of the Canadian Dental Association* 50: 363–8.

Ley, P. (1976) 'Towards better doctor–patient communication', in A. Bennett (ed.) *Communication Between Doctors and Patients*, London: Nuffield Provincial Hospitals Trust.

Ley, P. and Spelman, M. (1976) *Communicating With the Patient*, London: Staples Press.

Liddell, A. and May, B. (1984) 'Some characteristics of regular and irregular attenders for dental check-ups', *British Journal of Clinical Psychology* 23: 19–26.

Liddell, A. (1985) 'Children's reports of dental anxiety and efficacy relating to dental visits', *Canadian Psychology* 26: abstract no. 295.

Lindsay, S., Humphris, G. and Barnby, G. (1987) 'Expectations and preferences for routine dentistry in anxious adult patients', *British Dental Journal* 163: 120–4.

Linn, E. (1971) 'The dentist–patient relationship', in D. Richards and L. Cohen (eds) *Social Sciences and Dentistry: A Critical Bibliography*, The Hague: FDI/A. Sijthoff.

Linn, E. (1974) 'What patients don't know about preventive care', *Journal of Public Health Dentistry* 34: 39–41.

Linn, E. (1976) 'Teenagers' attitudes, knowledge and behaviours related to oral health', *Journal of the American Dental Association* 92: 946–51.

Locker, D. (1983) *Disability and Disadvantage: The Consequences of Chronic Illness*, London: Tavistock.

Locker, D. (1988) 'The symptom iceberg in dentistry: treatment-seeking in relation to oral and facial pain', *Journal of the Canadian Dental Association* (forthcoming).

Locker, D. and Grushka, M. (1987a) 'Prevalence of oral and facial pain and discomfort: preliminary results of a mail survey', *Community Dentistry and Oral Epidemiology* 15: 169–72.

Locker, D. and Grushka, M. (1987b) 'The impact of dental and facial pain', *Journal of Dental Research* 66: 1414–17.

Locker, D., Leake, J. and Schabas, R. (1987) 'The oral health status of persons aged 50 years and over in East York, Ontario', Faculty of Dentistry, University of Toronto, unpublished.

Locker, D. and Slade, M. (1988) 'The prevalence of symptoms of temporomandibular disorders', *Community Dentistry and Oral Epidemiology* (forthcoming).

Love, R. and Kalnins, I. (1984) 'Individualist and structuralist perspectives on nutrition education for Canadian children', *Social Science and Medicine* 18: 199–204.

McGrath, P., Veber, L. and Hearn, M. (1985) 'Multidimensional pain assessment in children', in H. Fields (ed.) *Advances in Pain Research and Therapy*, Vol. 9, New York: Raven Press.

MacIntyre, S. (1986) 'The patterning of health by social position in contemporary Britain: directions for sociological research', *Social Science and Medicine* 23: 393–415.

McKeown, T. (1979) *The Role of Medicine: Dream, Mirage or Nemesis?* Oxford: Blackwell Scientific.

McKinlay, J. (1972) 'Some approaches and problems in the study of the use of services: an overview', *Journal of Health and Social Behaviour* 13: 115–52.

McKinlay, J. (1973) 'Social networks, lay consultation and help-seeking behaviour', *Social Forces*, 53: 275–92.

McKinlay, J. (1974) 'A case for refocusing upstream — the political economy of ill-health', *Applying Behavioural Science to Cardiovascular Risk*, Proceedings of American Heart Foundation Conference, Seattle.

McKinlay, J. (1977) 'The business of good doctoring or doctoring as good business: reflections on Freidson's view of the medical game', *International Journal of Health Services* 7: 469–83.

McKinlay, J. and McKinlay, S. (1977) 'The questionable contribution of medical measures to the decline in mortality in the United States in the twentieth century', *Millbank Memorial Fund Quarterly* 55: 405–28.

MacMahon, B. and Pugh, T. (1970) *Epidemiological Principles and Methods*, Boston: Little, Brown & Co.

McPherson, B. (1983) *Aging as a Social Process*, Toronto: Butterworths.

Manga, P. and Charette, A. (1986) 'The patterns and determinants of the utilization of dental care services in Canada', *Canadian Journal of Public Health* 77, Supplement 1: 119–23.

Manga, P. (1987) 'Equality of access and inequalities in health status', in D. Coburn, C. D'Arcy, G. Torrance and P. New (eds) *Health and Canadian Society*, Markham, Ontario: Fitzhenry & Whiteside.

Manning, W., Bailit, H., Benjamin, B. and Newhouse, J. (1986) *The Demand for Dental Care: Evidence from a Randomised Trial in Health Insurance*, Santa Monica: Rand.

Marco, T. (1976) 'Periodontal emotional stress syndrome', *Journal of Periodontology*, 48: 67–8.

Markula, J., Murtomaa, H. and Anaimo, J. (1977) 'Conceptions of Finnish people about the etiology and prevention of dental caries and periodontal disorders', *Community Dentistry and Oral Epidemiology* 5: 108–13.

Mausner, J. and Kramer, S. (1985) *Epidemiology — An Introductory Text*, Philadelphia: W.B. Saunders.

Mechanic, D. (1968) *Medical Sociology*, New York: Free Press.

Melamed, B., Weinstein, D. and Hawes, R. (1975) 'Reduction of fear-related dental management using filmed modeling', *Journal of the American Dental Association* 90: 822–6.

Melzack, R. and Wall, P. (1965) 'Pain mechanisms: a new theory', *Science* 150: 971–9.

Melzack, R. (1973) *The Puzzle of Pain*, New York: Basic Books.

Merskey, H. and Spear, E. (1967) *Pain: Psychological and Psychiatric Aspects*, London: Baillière, Tindall & Cassell.

Meskin, L., Brown, J. and Brunelle, J. (1988) 'Patterns of edentulism in US working adults and senior citizens', *Journal of Dental Research* 67 (special issue): abstract no. 510.

Miller, J., Elwood, P. and Swallow, J. (1975) 'Dental pain: an incidence study', *British Dental Journal* 139: 327–8.

Miller, M., Murphy, P. and Miller, T. (1978) 'Comparison of electromyographic feedback and progressive relaxation training in treating circumscribed anxiety stress reactions', *Journal of Consulting and Clinical Psychology* 46: 1291–8.

Miller, S. and Firestone, J. (1947) 'Psychosomatic factors in the etiology of periodontal disease: a critical review of the literature', *American Journal of Orthodontics and Oral Surgery* 33: 672–5.

Miller, W. (1987) 'Does oral health influence quality of life?', *Gerodontics* 3: 99.

Moline, J. (1986) 'Professionals and professions: a philosophical examination of an ideal', *Social Science and Medicine* 22: 501–8.

Morgan, M. (1980) 'Marital status, health, illness and service use', *Social Science and Medicine* 14A: 633–43.

Murray, J. (1983) 'The changing pattern of dental disease and treatment', in J. Murray (ed.) *The Prevention of Dental Disease*, Oxford: Oxford University Press.

Murray, P. (1987) 'A longitudinal study of the contribution of dental experience of children between the ages of nine and twelve to their dental anxiety', MSc thesis, Memorial University of Newfoundland, unpublished.

Naidoo, J. (1986) 'Limits to individualism', in S. Rodmell and A. Watt (eds) *The Politics of Health Education*, London: Routledge & Kegan Paul.

National Centre for Health Services Research (1982) National Health Care Expenditure Study, *Prescribed Medicines: Use, Expenditures and Source of Payment*, PHS Publication no. 82–3320, Hyattsville, Maryland.

National Centre for Health Statistics (1987) *Health, United States, 1986*, Department of Health and Human Services Publication No. (PHS) 87–1232.

Navarro, V. (1976) *Medicine Under Capitalism*, Beckenham: Croom Helm.

Nichols, S., Waters, W., Fraser, J., Wheeler, M. and Ingham, S. (1981) 'Delay in the presentation of breast symptoms for consultant investigations', *Community Medicine* 3: 217–25.

Nikias, M. (1985) 'Oral disease and the quality of life', *American Journal of Public Health* 75, 11–12.

Nikias, M., Bailit, H., Beck, J., Cohen, L. K., Conrad, D., Giddon, D., Reisine, S. and Sheiham, A. (1979) *Progress Report to the WHO/Oral Research Advisory Group*, unpublished.

Nikias, M., Fink, R. and Shapiro, S. (1975) 'Comparisons of poverty and non-poverty groups on dental status, needs and practices', *Journal of Public Health Dentistry* 35: 237–58.

Nikias, M., Fink, R. and Sollecito, W. (1977) 'Oral health status in relation to socioeconomic and ethnic characteristics of urban adults in the USA', *Community Dentistry and Oral Epidemiology* 5: 200–6.

Nuttall, N. (1985) 'Financial implications of the 1985 GDS patient charging system', *British Dental Journal* 159: 375–6.

OPCS (1978) *Occupational Mortality, Decennial Supplement 1970–2, England and Wales*, London: HMSO.

OPCS (1985) *Population Projections 1985–2025*, London: HMSO.

OPCS (1986) 'The 1983 update on adult dental health from OPCS', *British Dental Journal* 160: 246–53.

OPCS (1987) *Population Projections 1985–2025*, London: HMSO.

O'Mullane, D. and Robinson, M. (1977) 'The distribution of dentists and the uptake of dental treatment by schoolchildren in England', *Community Dentistry and Oral Epidemiology* 5: 156–9.

O'Shea, R., Corah, N. and Thines, T. (1986) 'Dental patients' advice on how to reduce anxiety', *General Dentistry* 15: 44–7.

O'Shea, R., Corah, N. and Ayer, W. (1984) 'Sources of dentists' stress', *Journal of the American Dental Association* 109: 48–51.

Orner, G. (1976) *Mortality Study of Dentists: Final Report*, National Institute of Safety and Health, Temple University.

Oulette, P. (1978) 'Psychological ramifications of facial change in relation to orthodontic treatment and orthognathic surgery', *Journal of Oral Surgery* 36: 787–90.

Page, R. (1984) 'Periodontal diseases in the elderly: a critical evalutation of current information', *Gerodontology* 3: 63–71.

Palmer, S., Wiggins, R. and Bewley, B. (1980) 'Infant deaths in inner London: a health care planning team study', *Community Medicine* 2: 102–8.

Parsons, T. (1951) *The Social System*, Glencoe: Free Press.

Patrick, D. (1982) 'The measurement of health', in D. Patrick and G. Scambler (eds) *Sociology As Applied to Medicine*, London: Baillière Tindall.

Patrick, D., Darby, S., Green, S., Horton, G., Locker, D. and Wiggins, R. (1981) 'Screening for disability in the inner city', *Journal of Epidemiology and Community Health* 35: 65–70.

Pearse, I. and Crocker, L. (1949) *The Peckham Experiment*, London: Allen & Unwin.

Peter, J. and Chinsky, R. (1974) 'Sociological aspects of cleft palate adults I: marriage', *Cleft Palate Journal* 11, 259–309.

Peterkin, B., Rizek, R., Posati, L. and Harris, S. (1987) 'When, where, with whom and what older Americans eat', *Gerodontics* 3: 14–19.

Plaja, A. and Cohen, S. (1968) 'Communications with physicians and patients in outpatient clinics: social and cultural factors', *Millbank Memorial Fund Quarterly* 46: 161–213.

Powell, M. and Eccles, J. (1970) 'The health and work of two professional groups: dentists and pharmacists', *Dental Practitioner* 20: 373–6.

Powles, J. (1973) 'On the limitations of modern medicine', *Science, Medicine and Man* 1: 31–48.

Ranta, K., Tuominen, R. and Paunio, I. (1987) 'Perceived oral health status and ability to chew among an adult Finnish population', *Gerodontics* 3: 136–9.

Rayner, J. (1970) 'Socioeconomic status and factors influencing the dental health practices of mothers', *American Journal of Public Health* 60: 1250–8.

Reisine, S. (1984) 'The economic, social and psychological impact of oral health conditions, diseases and treatments', in L. Cohen and P. Bryant (eds) *Social Sciences and Dentistry: A Critical Bibliography*, London: FDI/Quintessence.

Reisine, S. (1985) 'Dental health and public policy: the social impact of dental disease', *American Journal of Public Health* 75: 27–30.

Reisine, S. and Miller, J. (1986) 'A longitudinal study of work loss related to dental diseases', *Social Science and Medicine* 22: 1309–14.

Rise, J. (1985) 'Evalution of social inequality of use of dental services in Norway', *Community Dentistry and Oral Epidemiology* 13: 57–60.

Rosenstock, I. (1966) 'Why people use health services', *Millbank Memorial Fund Quarterly* 44: 94–127.

Rugh, J., Jacobs, D., Taverna, D. and Johnston, W. (1984) 'Psychophysiological changes and oral conditions', in L. Cohen and P. Bryant (eds) *Social Sciences and Dentistry: A Critical Bibliography*, London: FDI/Quintessence.

Rugh, J. and Solberg, W. (1974) 'Cognitive components of masseter muscle exercise for bruxism subjects', *Journal of Dental Research* 53: abstract no. 464, 170.

Scambler, A., Scambler, G. and Craig, D. (1981) 'Kinship and friendship networks and women's demand for primary medical care', *Journal of the Royal College of General Practitioners* 26: 746–50.

Schoen, M. (1985) 'Does dentistry as we know it have a future?', *Journal of Public Health Dentistry* 45: 130–3.

Schou, L. (1985) 'Active involvement principle in dental health education', *Community Dentistry and Oral Epidemiology* 13: 128–32.

Scrivens, E., Cunningham, D., Charlton, J. and Holland, W. (1985) 'Measuring the impact of health interventions: a review of available instruments', *Effective Health Care* 2, 247–59.

Segal, H. (1986) 'Categories of emergency patient', *General Dentistry* 34: 37–42.

Selye, H. (1956) *The Stress of Life*, New York: McGraw-Hill.

Selye, H. (1974) *Stress Without Distress*, Philadelphia: J. B. Lippincott Co.

Sharpenak, A., Bobyleva, V. and Gorozhankina, L. (1963) 'Role of protein, lysine, certain mineral substances and vitamins A and D in prevention of dental caries', *Stomatologia* 42: 7–12.

Shaw, O. (1975) 'Dental anxiety in children', *British Dental Journal* 139: 134–9.

Shaw, W., Meek, S. and Jones, D. (1980a) 'Nicknames, teasing, harassment and the salience of dental features among school children', *British Journal of Orthodontics* 7: 75–80.

Shaw, W., Addy, M. and Ray, C. (1980b) 'Dental and social effects of malocclusion and effectiveness of orthodontic treatment: a review', *Community Dentistry and Oral Epidemiology* 8: 36–45.

Sheiham, A. and Croog, S. (1981) 'The psychosocial impact of dental diseases on individuals and communities', *Journal of Behavioral Medicine* 4, 257–72.

Sheiham, A., Maizels, J. and Cushing, A. (1982) 'The concept of need in dentistry', *International Dental Journal* 32: 265–8.

Skipper, J. and Leonard, R. (1968) 'Children, stress and hospitalisation: a field experiment', *Journal of Health and Social Behaviour* 9: 275–87.

Smith, J. and Sheiham, A. (1979) 'How dental conditions handicap the elderly', *Community Dentistry and Oral Epidemiology* 7: 305–10.

Smith, J., Steele, L. and Sheiham, A. (1983) 'Delivery programmes for elderly and isolated populations', *International Dental Journal* 33: 301–7.

Solberg, W., Woo, M. and Houston, J. (1979) 'Prevalence of mandibular dysfunction in young adults', *Journal of the American Dental Association* 98: 25–34.

Speculand, B., Hughes, A. and Goss, A. (1984) 'Role of recent stressful life events experience in the onset of TMJ dysfunction pain', *Community Dentistry and Oral Epidemiology* 12: 197–202.

Speller, V. (1985) 'Defining health promotion', *Health Education Journal* 44: 96–7.

Spencer, A. (1980) 'The estimation of need for dental care', *Journal of Public Health Dentistry* 40: 311–27.

Starr, P. (1978) 'Self-esteem and behavioral functioning of teenagers with oro-facial clefts', *Rehabilitation Literature* 39: 233–5.

Stein, S., Loft, G., Davis, H. and Hart, D. (1982) 'Symptoms of TMJ dysfunction as related to stress measured by the Social Readjustment Rating Scale', *Journal of Prosthetic Dentistry* 47: 545–8.

Steinman, R. (1960) 'The effect of stress upon the incidence of dental caries', *Journal of the California State Dental Association* 28: 367–71.

Steinman, R., Mothersill, K. and Brooke, R. (1961) 'Comparison of caries incidence in exercised and immobilised rats', *Journal of Dental Research* 40: 218–23.

Stewart, M. (1984) 'What is a successful doctor–patient interview?', *Social Science and Medicine* 19: 167–75.

Stimson, G. and Webb, B. (1975) *Going to See the Doctor: The Consultation Process in General Practice*, London: Routledge & Kegan Paul.

Strayer, M., DiAngelis, A. and Loupe, M. (1986) 'Dentists' knowledge of aging in relation to perceived elderly patient behaviour', *Gerodontics* 2: 223–7.

Striffler, D. (1983) 'Dental treatment, need, demand and utilization', in D. Striffler, W. Young and B. Burt, *Dentistry, Dental Practice and the Community*, Philadelphia: W. B. Saunders.

Sutton, P. (1965) 'The early onset of acute dental caries following mental stress', *New York State Dental Journal* 31: 450–5.

Sutton, P. (1966) 'Stress and dental caries', in P. Staples (ed.) *Advances in Oral Biology*, New York: Academic Press.

Szasz, T. (1961) *The Myth of Mental Illness*, New York: Hocber/Harper.

Szasz, T. and Hollender, M. (1956) 'A contribution to the philosophy of medicine', *AMA Archives of Internal Medicine XVII* 97: 585–92.

Szwejda, L. (1960) 'Observed differences in total caries experience among white children of various socio-economic groups', *Public Health Dentistry* 20: 59–66.

Szwejda, L. (1962) 'Dental caries experience by race and socioeconomic level after eleven years of water fluoridation in Charlotte, North Carolina', *Public Health Dentistry* 22: 91–8.

Tala, A. and Ainamo, J. (1982) 'Changes in general behaviour and environmental factors related to dental health', in A. Frandsen (ed.) *Dental Health Care in Scandinavia*, Chicago: Quintessence.

Tamir, L. (1979) *Communication and the Aging Process*, New York: Pergamon Press.

Tan, H., Rutter, E. and Verhey, H. (1981) 'Effect of repeated dental health care education on gingival health, knowledge, attitudes, behaviour and perception', *Community Dentistry and Oral Epidemiology* 9: 15–21.

Tedesco, L., Keffer, M., Fleck-Kandath, C., Johannson, J., Christofferson, L., Albino, J. and Genco, R. (1988) 'Cognitions and oral health behaviour reports', *Journal of Dental Research* 67 (special issue): abstract no. 1321.

Thomas, L., Tiber, N. and Schireson, S. (1973) 'The effects of anxiety and frustration on muscular tension related to the temporomandibular joint syndrome', *Oral Surgery* 37: 763–9.

Thrash, W., Marr, J. and Box, T. (1982) 'Continuous self-monitoring of discomfort in the dental chair and feedback to the dentist', *Journal of Behavioural Assessment* 4: 273–84.

Todd, J. and Dodd, T. (1985) *Children's Dental Health in the United Kingdom, 1983*, London: HMSO.

Todd, J. and Walker, M. (1980) *Adult Dental Health: Vol. 1, England and Wales, 1968–78*, London: HMSO.

Todd, J., Walker, A. and Dodd, P. (1982) *Adult Dental Health: Vol. 2, United Kingdom, 1978*, London: HMSO.

Townsend, P. and Davidson, N. (1982) *Inequalities in Health: The Black Report*, Harmondsworth: Penguin.

Troxler, R. (1986) 'Human stress response and its possible relationship to disease', *Dental Clinics of North America* 30: S11–S27.

Tuckett, D., Boulton, M., Olson, C. and Williams, A. (1985) *Meetings Between Experts*, London: Tavistock.

US Department of Health and Human Services, Public Health Services (1981) *Focal Points* 22: 119–25.

US Department of Health and Human Services, Public Health Service, National Institute of Health (1987) *Oral Health of United States Adults: The National Survey of Oral Health in US Employed Adults and Seniors 1985–6*, NIH Publication no. 87–2868.

US Department of Health Education and Welfare (1979) *Health Status of Minorities and Low Income Groups*, DHEW Publication no. (HRA) 79–627. Washington: US Government Printing Office.

Uddenberg, M. (1979) 'Childbirth pain', in D. Osborne, M. Gruneberg and J. Eiser (eds) *Research in Psychology and Medicine 1*, London: Academic Press.

Venham, L. (1979) 'The effect of mother's presence on child's responses to dental treatment', *Journal of Dentistry for Children* 46: 219–75.

Verkleij, H. and Spruit, I. (1984) 'Selecting a health indicator for comparative health surveys', *Effective Health Care* 1: 251–6.

Wadsworth, M., Butterfield, W. and Blaney, H. (1971) *Health and Illness: The Choice of Treatment*, London: Tavistock.

Wall, P. and Ayer, W. (1984) 'Work loss among practicing dentists', *Journal of the American Dental Association* 108: 81–3.

Walsh, M. (1985) 'Effects of school-based health education on knowledge, attitudes and behavior of adolescents in San Francisco', *Community Dentistry and Oral Epidemiology* 13: 143–7.

Wardle, J. (1982a) 'Management of dental pain', paper presented at the British Psychological Society Conference.

Wardle, J. (1982b) 'Fear of dentistry', *British Journal of Medical Psychology* 55: 119–26.

Weddell, J. and Klein, A. (1981) 'Socio-economic correlation in oral disease in six- to thirty-six-month children', *American Academy of Paedodontics* 3: 306–10.

Weinstein, P. (1982) 'Humanistic application of behavioral strategies in oral hygiene instruction', *Clinical Preventive Dentistry* 4: 15–19.

Weinstein, P., Getz, T. and Milgrom, P. (1983) 'Oral self care: a promising alternative behavioral model', *Journal of the American Dental Association* 107: 67–70.

Weinstein, P., Getz, T. and Milgrom, P. (1985) *Oral Self Care: Strategies for Preventive Dentistry*, Reston: Reston Publishing Company.

Weinstein, P., Milgrom, P., Ratenar, P., Read, W. and Morrison, K. (1978) 'Dentists' perceptions of their patients', *Journal of Public Health Dentistry* 38: 10–21.

Weintraub, J. and Burt, B. (1985) 'Oral health status in the US: tooth loss and edentulism', *Journal of Dental Education* 49: 368–76.

Weisenberg, J., Kegeles, S. and Lund, K. (1980) 'Children's health beliefs and acceptance of a preventive dental activity', *Journal of Health and Social Behaviour* 21: 59–72.

WHO (1980) *International Classification of Impairments, Disabilities and Handicaps*, Geneva: World Health Organisation.

Wilensky, H. (1964) 'The professionalization of everyone?', *American Journal of Sociology* 119: 68–79.

Wilkins, R. and Adams, O. (1983) *Healthfulness of Life*, Montreal: Institute for Research on Public Policy.

Williamson, J. (1964) 'Old people at home: their unreported needs', *The Lancet* 3: 1117–20.

Winer, G. (1982) 'A review and analysis of children's fearful behaviour in dental settings', *Child Development* 53: 1111–31.

Wolf, S. (1959) 'The pharmacology of placebos', *Pharmacological Review* 11: 689–705.

Wood, P. (1980) 'The language of disablement: a glossary relating to disease and its consequences', *International Journal of Rehabilitation* 2: 86–92.

Wotman, S. and Goldman, H. (1982) 'Pressures on the dental care system in the United States', *American Journal of Public Health* 72: 684–9.

Zborowski, M. (1952) 'Cultural components in responses to pain', *Journal of Social Issues* 8: 16–30.

Zola, I. (1966) 'Culture and symptoms: an analysis of patients' presenting complaints', *American Sociological Review* 31: 615–30.

Zola, I. (1973) 'Pathways to the doctor: from person to patient', *Social Science and Medicine* 7: 677–89.

Zola, I. (1975) 'In the name of health and illness', *Social Science and Medicine* 9: 83–7.

Name index

Subject index